Wilderness First Aid Made Easy - 2022 Edition

ISBN: 978-1-7335440-9-2

Wilderness First Aid Made Easy is an independent publication and has not been authorized, sponsored or otherwise approved by the owners of the trademarks or the service marks referenced in this product. This publication has been designed as a companion resource for individuals who have attended a Wilderness First Aid (WFA) certification course and hold a WFA certification.

The procedures and protocols in this book are based on the most current recommendations of responsible medical sources. The author and the publisher, however, make no guarantee as to, and assume no responsibility for, the correctness, sufficiency or completeness of such information or recommendations. Furthermore, the author and the publisher do not assume and hereby disclaim any liability for loss, damage, injury or disruption caused by errors, or omissions, whether such omissions result from negligence, accident or any other cause. Other or additional safety measures may be required under particular circumstances. Use of this publication does not create a physician-patient relationship. You are solely responsible for your decision to obtain treatment from a medical professional.

This publication is designed for educational purposes only and not for the purpose of rendering medical advice. The information presented through this publication is not intended to replace the counsel of a physician. It is not intended as a statement of the standards of care required in any particular situation, because circumstances and the patient's physical condition can vary widely from one emergency to another. Nor is it intended that this book shall in any way advise people responding to emergency situations concerning legal authority to perform the activities or procedures discussed.

Introduction - A

A Wilderness First Aid (WFA) Course is one of the most intensive first aid courses a person can attend. The course takes place over two days with 16 to 20 hours of instruction. WFA students are taught many of the basic life support concepts as taught in a 16-week emergency medical technician courses. WFA students learn the primary and secondary patient assessment, how to identify and treat patient injuries and illnesses, how to reduce and splint fractures and how to care for a patient for up to several days while awaiting rescue.

The WFA Certification course is intense. So much information is covered in such a short period of time that many students comment that attending a Wilderness First Aid course is like drinking from a fire hose and attempting not to drown.

When I was a WFA student, I spent most of the course heads-down, furiously writing notes. We sat for lectures and then immediately participated in scenarios switching off roles of playing patient and caregiver. My scribbled notes were used in the hands-on scenarios to practice what was just taught a few minutes prior. I felt rushed and overwhelmed. At the end of day one, my brain was fried.

At the end of day two, I graduated with a sense of accomplishment that successfully I earned my Wilderness First Aid certification, but I wondered how competent I was after two intensive days of training with no time to absorb what I learned. I began searching for a solution that will enable me to review, refresh and retain what I learned during the two-day class.

A few years prior to earning my WFA certification, I read Checklist Manifesto, by Dr. Atul Gawande. Checklist Manifesto is a book that details the use of checklists in healthcare. The author is a surgeon and he began experimenting with using checklists in hospitals. The results of his research were astonishing. Dr. Gawande found that for doctors and nurses that used checklists, the consistency of care improved to the point where the average length of patient stay in intensive care dropped by half. In another example where a hospital implemented a handwashing checklist and empowering any nurse from stopping a surgeon from treating a patient if they missed any items on the checklist, in just one year, the infection rate went from eleven percent to zero.

One of my favorite quotes from Checklist Manifesto -

"Whether running to the store to buy ingredients for a cake, preparing an airplane for takeoff, or evaluating a sick person in the hospital, if you miss just one key thing, you might as well not have made the effort at all."

Gawande, Atul. The Checklist Manifesto: How to Get Things Right. London: Profile Books, 2011. Page 36.

Missing one step in the Patient Assessment may overlook bleeding the caregiver does not see. Not checking the airway correctly, missing checking for circulation in an extremity or not recognizing sepsis in a patient could result in negative patient outcomes and even death.

I was training to become a certified Wilderness First Aid instructor and part of the training involved attending the two-day WFA course six times over a four-month period. During this time of training, I converted the entire WFA course into approximately forty checklists.
I discovered that checklists have limitations as they do not illustrate decision flow and they do not function well when there are multiple decision points. In first aid, there are many decision points and these decision points add complexity to text-based checklists.

So, I went one step further and I converted my checklists to "medical algorithms." You may not be familiar with medical algorithms, but they are used in healthcare to improve and standardize decisions made in the delivery of medical care. Medical algorithms assist in the selection and application of treatment. I found that medical algorithms are able to reduce hundreds of pages of text into step-by-step checklists that are displayed in sequential order and include "yes-no" decision nodes that graphically illustrate the entire patient care process. Medical algorithms make refreshing our knowledge easier because each step of the patient care process is visually illustrated.

I created Wilderness First Aid medical algorithms to help me refresh my memory and stay current on my knowledge. I regularly reviewed the algorithms, and it was not long until I achieved fluency in emergency first aid care. In 2019 I published these algorithms in my first book, Emergency First Aid Care Flow Diagrams - Wilderness First Aid Edition. My book became a standard handout to all of the students attending my WFA classes. I used the algorithms to teach each section of the WFA course and the benefits of using algorithms in my classes became evident.

The 2022 edition of this book includes QR Codes that you can scan with your smartphone and view over fifty presentations and demonstrations from my Wilderness First Aid Course. I believe you will find the integration of textbook and video resources to be an excellent learning and knowledge refreshment tool.

My education in emergency first aid did not end with my WFA certification. I went on to become a state-licensed Emergency Medical Technician, a National Registry Emergency Medical Technician, a Wilderness Emergency Medical Technician, a Level II NFPA 1041 instructor and an American Red Cross Instructor-Trainer. I am certified as a Wilderness First Aid Instructor and a Wilderness First Responder Instructor for the American Red Cross, the American Safety and Health Institute and the Emergency Care and Safety Institute.

My life passion is to educate people with no medical background on how to provide first aid in a medical emergency and continue to provide care while waiting on EMS to arrive.

Wilderness First Aid Made Easy will help you to remember the steps in patient assessment and care. During a Wilderness First Aid course, this book will reduce the time you spend taking notes and allow you to concentrate on the lectures. After earning your certification, this book will enable you to keep your knowledge fresh by serving you as an excellent review tool.

Jeffrey S. Imel WEMT, NREMT
October 2021

A Wilderness First Aid (WFA) Course is one of the most intensive first aid courses a person can attend. The course takes place over two days with 16 to 20 hours of instruction. WFA students are taught many of the basic life support concepts as taught in a 16-week emergency medical technician courses. WFA students learn the primary and secondary patient assessment, how to identify and treat patient injuries and illnesses, how to reduce and splint fractures and how to care for a patient for up to several days while awaiting rescue.

The WFA Certification course is serious. So much information is covered in such a short period of time that many students comment that attending a Wilderness First Aid course is like drinking from a fire hose and attempting not to drown.

When I was a WFA student, I spent most of the course heads-down, furiously writing notes. We sat for lectures and then immediately participated in scenarios switching off roles of playing patient and caregiver. My scribbled notes were used in the hands-on scenarios to practice what was just taught a few minutes prior. I felt rushed and overwhelmed. At the end of day one, my brain was fried.

At the end of day two, I graduated with a sense of accomplishment that successfully I earned my Wilderness First Aid certification, but I wondered how competent I was after two intensive days of training with no time to absorb what I learned. I began searching for a solution that will enable me to review, refresh and retain what I learned during the two-day class.

A few years prior to earning my WFA certification, I read *Checklist Manifesto*, by Dr. Atul Gawande. *Checklist Manifesto* is a book that details the use of checklists in healthcare. The author is a surgeon and he began experimenting with using checklists in hospitals. The results of his research were astonishing. Dr. Gawande found that for doctors and nurses that used checklists, the consistency of care improved to the point where the average length of patient stay in intensive care dropped by half. In another example where a hospital implemented a handwashing checklist and empowering any nurse from stopping a surgeon from treating a patient if they missed any items on the checklist, in just one year, the infection rate went from eleven percent to zero.

One of my favorite quotes from *Checklist Manifesto* -

> *"Whether running to the store to buy ingredients for a cake, preparing an airplane for takeoff, or evaluating a sick person in the hospital, if you miss just one key thing, you might as well not have made the effort at all."*
>
> - Gawande, Atul. The Checklist Manifesto: How to Get Things Right. London: Profile Books, 2011. Page 36.

Missing one step in the Patient Assessment may overlook bleeding the caregiver does not see. Not checking the airway correctly, missing checking for circulation in an extremity or not recognizing sepsis in a patient could result in negative patient outcomes and even death.

I was training to become a certified Wilderness First Aid instructor and part of the training involved attending the two-day WFA course six times over a four-month period. During this time of training, I converted the entire WFA course into approximately forty checklists.

I discovered that checklists have limitations as they do not illustrate decision flow and they do not function well when there are multiple decision points. In first aid, there are many decision points and these decision points add complexity to text-based checklists.

How to Use Algorithms - B

The algorithms in this book will walk you step-by-step through the patient care process. These algorithms are "work flow" diagrams for identifying and treating illnesses and injuries austere environments.

How to Navigate the Algorithms

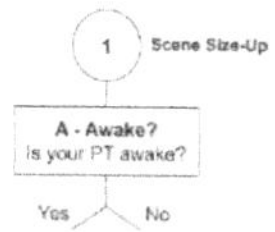

Start on Page 1 – Scene Size-Up in the upper left-hand corner and follow the diagram. All algorithms begin in the upper left-hand corner and end at the bottom or the bottom right-hand corner.

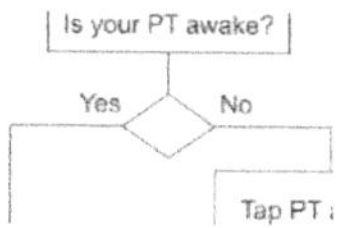

You will come to diamond shape junctions in the algorithms that will require you to answer a Yes – No question. Answer the question and continue to follow the diagram. Follow the instructions found in each box and answer the Yes-No questions. The algorithms will enable you to identify and treat the most common injuries and illness found in austere environments.

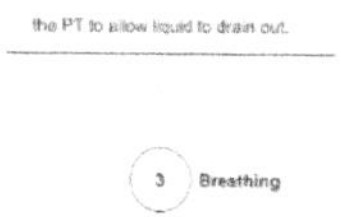

The algorithms will lead you to a circle with a number at the bottom or the right side of the page. The circle indicates what page you should proceed to next. Go to the indicated page and start the algorithm on the upper left-hand side,

Evacuation Guidelines.

You will find Suggested Evacuation Guidelines throughout Wilderness First Aid Made Easy. The guidelines offer suggestions based on Wilderness Medical Society Guidelines and Boy Scout of America Guidelines. However, these are only suggestions. You should always err on the side a safety and evacuate anytime your intuition is telling you to evacuate immediately.

Sample Scenarios

The following two sample scenarios will illustrate how to use the algorithms to identify and treat both life threatening and non-life threatening illnesses and injuries.

Scenario: A person in the group you are leading on a hike is complaining of stomach nausea and does not feel like eating.

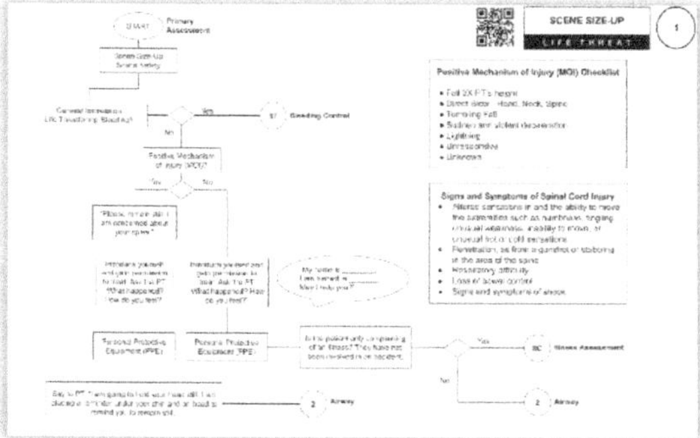

Page 1 Scene Size-Up
The patient is complaining of an illness and is not injured and no possible Positive Mechanism of Injury. The scene is safe. **Go to Page 8 – Illness Assessment**. Document care using a SOAP Note.

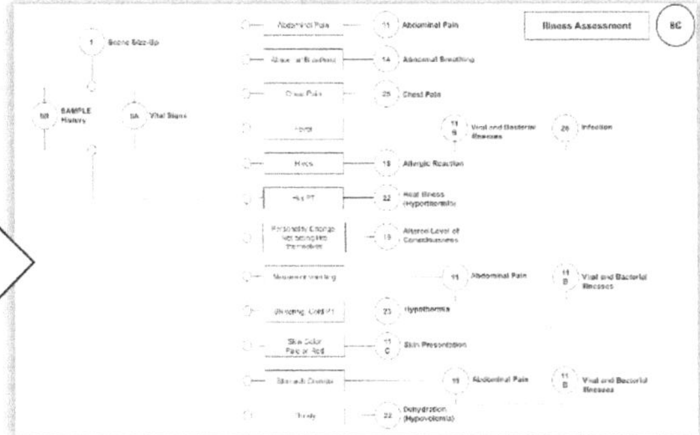

Page 8 – Illness Assessment
Collect the patient's SAMPLE History and a set of Vital Signs.

SAMPLE History
Signs and Symptoms – Stomach nausea and no appetite
Allergies – Penicillin
Medications – None
Past Medical History – None
Last In/Last Out
Water all day from canteen – trusted source
Breakfast (Toast) seven hours ago at home.
Refuses to eat lunch. Patient is not hungry.
Pee – 30 minutes ago. Clear.
Poop – 30 minutes ago. Runny. Not normal.

SAMPLE History Highlights
- Stomach nausea and no appetite
- Poop – Runny. Not normal.

Vital Signs Highlights
- Skin is Pale, Cool and Moist

Vital Signs
Time: 2:00 PM
LOC: A+Ox3
HR: 74
RR: 14
Skin: Pale, Cool, Moist

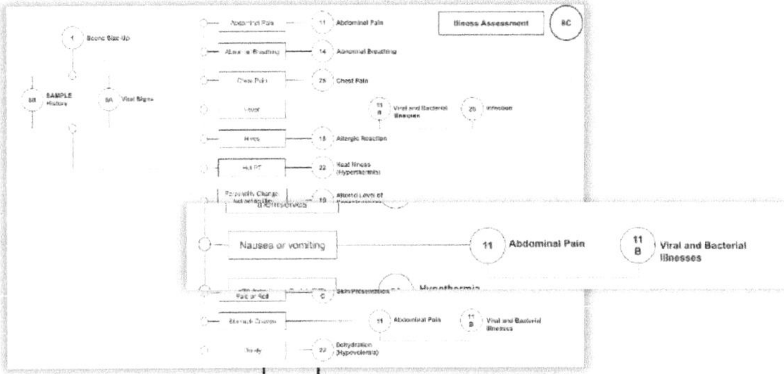

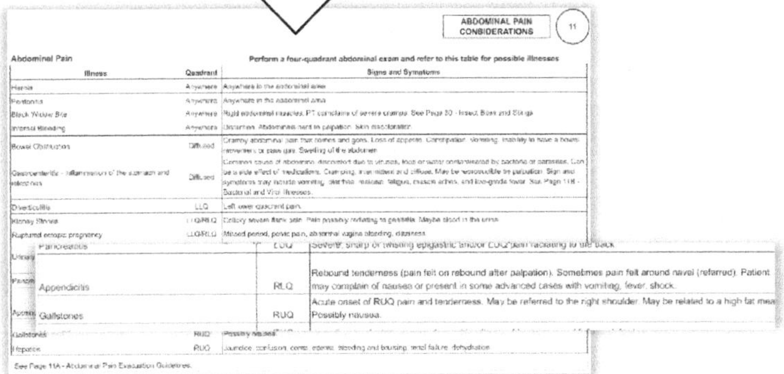

Go to Page 8C – Illness Assessment.
Look up the symptoms of stomach nausea.
Go to Page 11 – Abdominal Pain

Page 11 – Abdominal Pain
Perform a Four-Quadrant Abdominal Exam. The patient complains of rebound tenderness on palpation of the Right Lower Quadrant (RLQ).

The patient is presenting with the signs and symptoms of appendicitis.

See Page 11A for Evacuation Guidelines. The patient requires immediate evacuation to the hospital.

Scenario: A person in the group you are leading fell on the trail and is complaining of severe lower left leg pain.

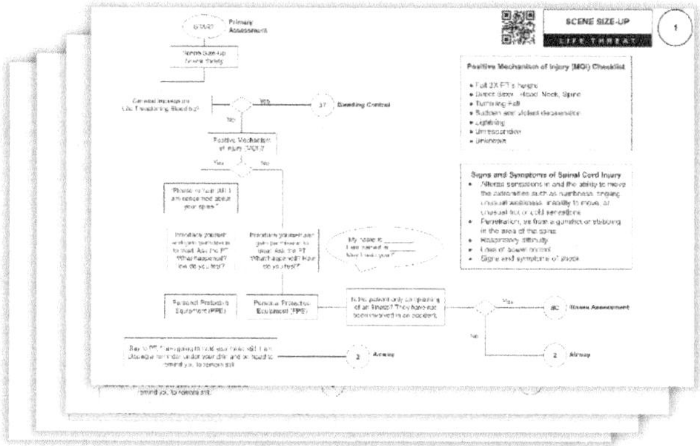

Complete the entire **Primary Assessment Pages 1 – 7**. You find no life threatening injuries or illnesses. You find the patient's lower left leg is painful to palpation and movement. You see a bruise on the patient's lower left shin at the pain site, indicating a possible bone fracture to the lower left leg.

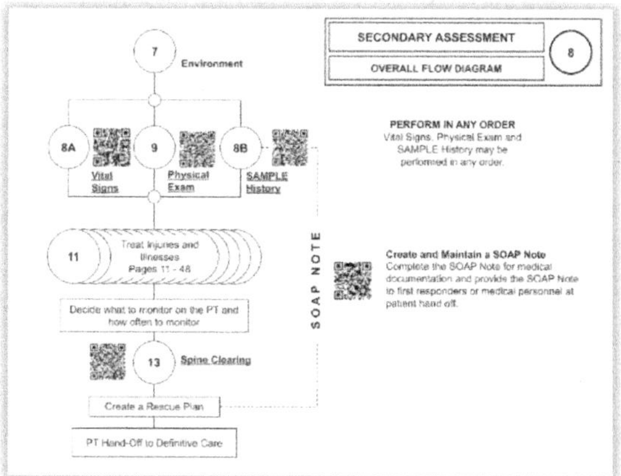

Complete the **entire Secondary Assessment Pages 8 – 10.** You find no other injuries or illnesses. The patient is presenting with the signs and symptoms of a bone fracture in the lower left leg. Document care using a SOAP Note.

SAMPLE History
Signs and Symptoms – Lower left leg pain on palpation and movement. Bruise at pain site.
Allergies – Seasonal
Medications – Allegra
Past Medical History – None
Last In/Last Out
- Water all day from canteen – trusted source
- Lunch one hour ago. Peanut butter sandwich from home.
- Pee – 30 minutes ago. Clear.
- Poop – This morning. Normal.

SAMPLE History Highlights
Lower left leg pain on palpation and movement. Bruise at pain site.

Vital Signs Highlights
- Normal

Vital Signs
Time: 1:30 PM
LOC: A+Ox3
HR: 70
RR: 12
Skin: Pink, Warm, Dry

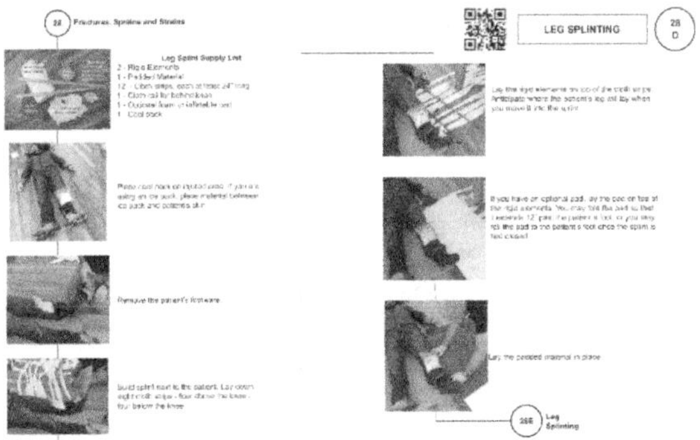

Treat the patient's injuries. Apply a leg splint to the patient's left leg using the **Leg Splinting** checklists on **Pages 28D – 28F.**

Create a rescue plan and evacuate the patient to definitive medical care.

How to Navigate the Algorithms

Start on page one and follow the algorithms, answering the "Yes-No" questions. The algorithms start in the upper left hand corner of each page and end at the bottom of each page at a circle with a page number, indicating the next page you should proceed to continue care.

QR Codes found on each page of the book provide an explanation of each page plus demonstrations of the concepts being taught.

The algorithms will lead you through the entire patient assessment process and guide you in patient illness and injury identification and treatment for the most commonly encountered first aid emergencies in the outdoors.

OVERALL WFA CARE FLOW DIAGRAM

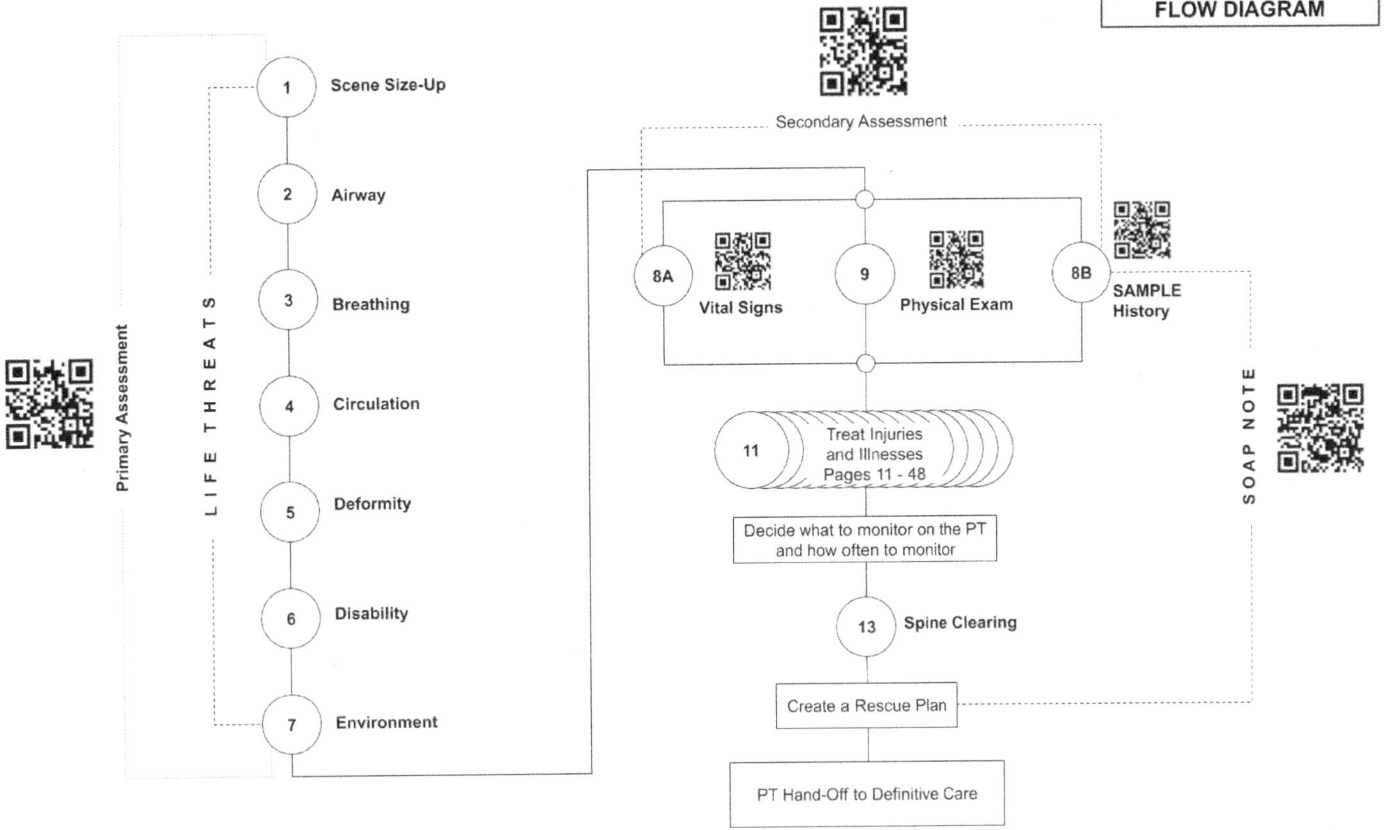

SCENE SIZE-UP

LIFE THREAT

1

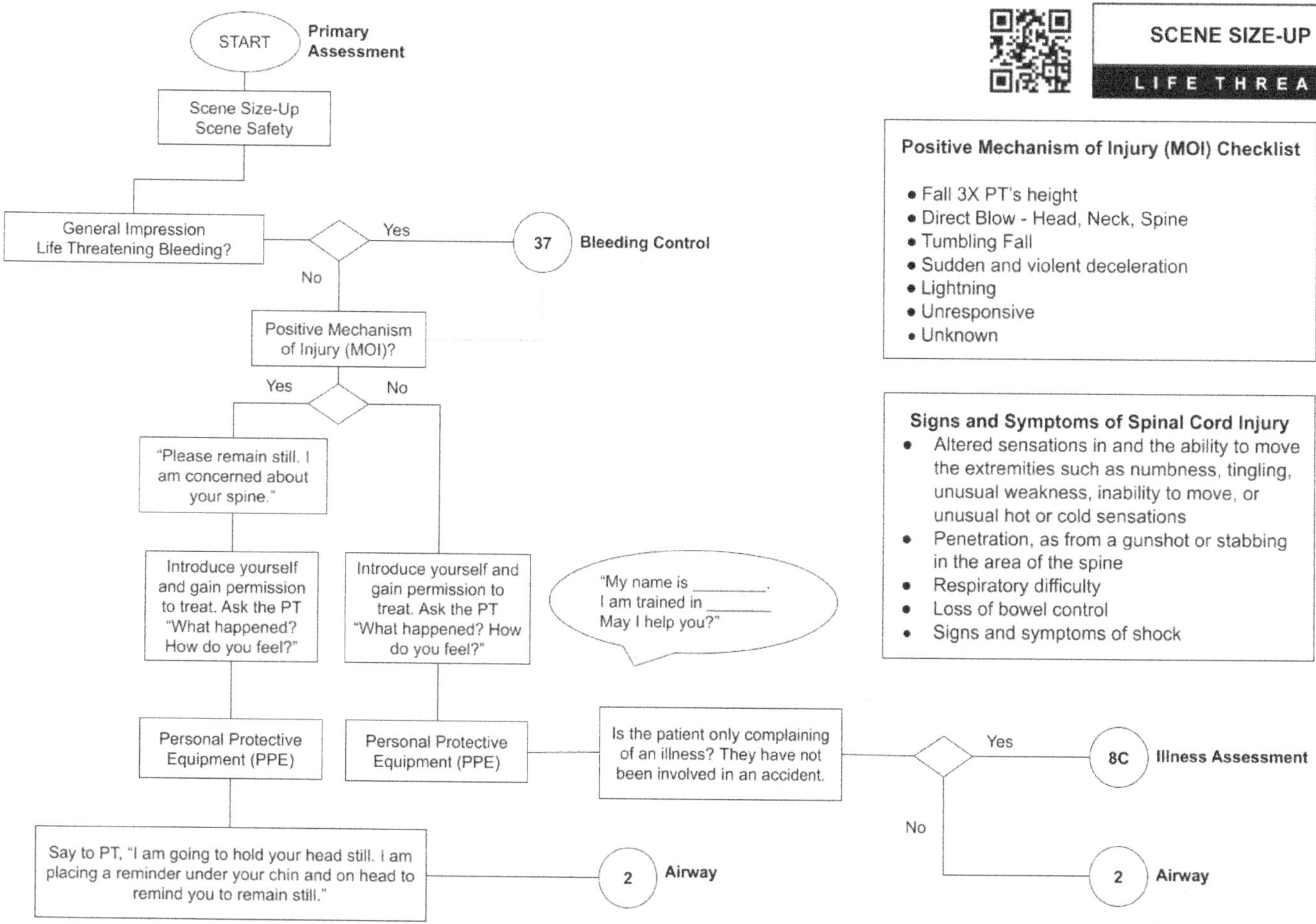

Positive Mechanism of Injury (MOI) Checklist

- Fall 3X PT's height
- Direct Blow - Head, Neck, Spine
- Tumbling Fall
- Sudden and violent deceleration
- Lightning
- Unresponsive
- Unknown

Signs and Symptoms of Spinal Cord Injury

- Altered sensations in and the ability to move the extremities such as numbness, tingling, unusual weakness, inability to move, or unusual hot or cold sensations
- Penetration, as from a gunshot or stabbing in the area of the spine
- Respiratory difficulty
- Loss of bowel control
- Signs and symptoms of shock

AIRWAY

LIFE THREAT

2

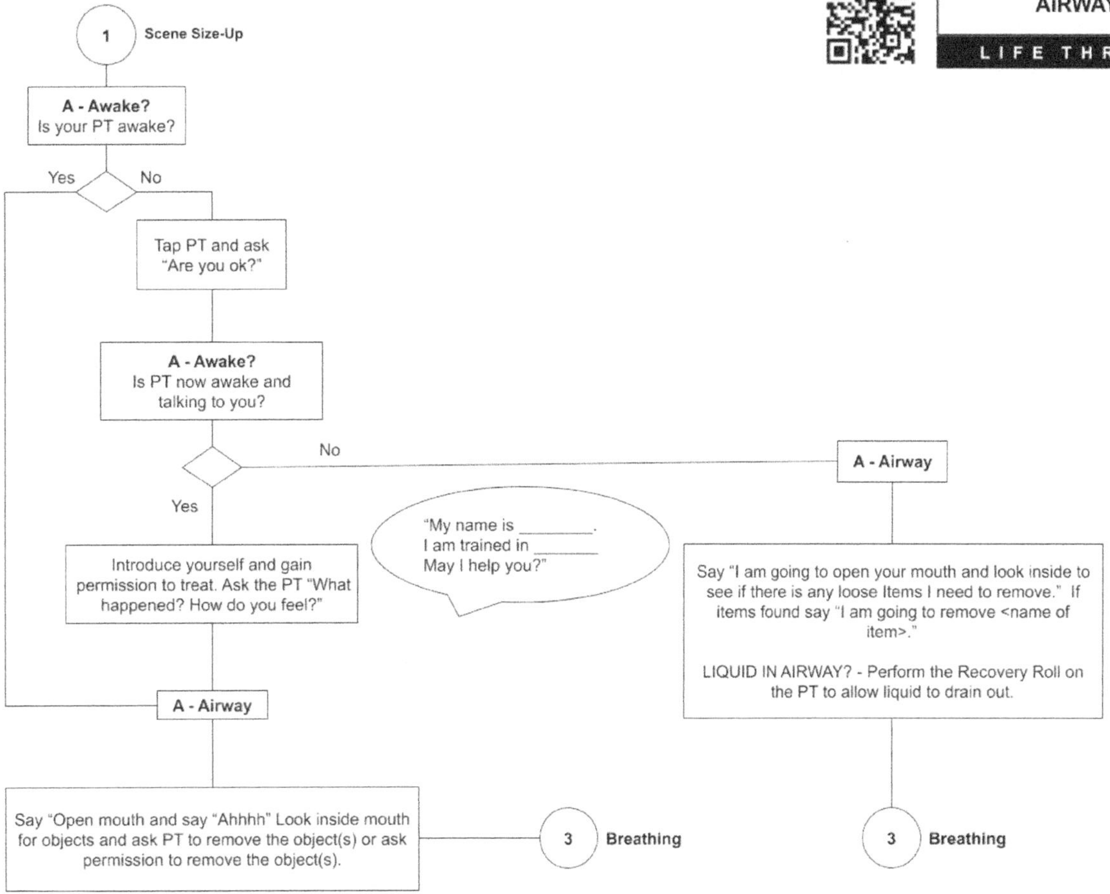

Recovery Roll Demonstration

BREATHING

LIFE THREAT

3

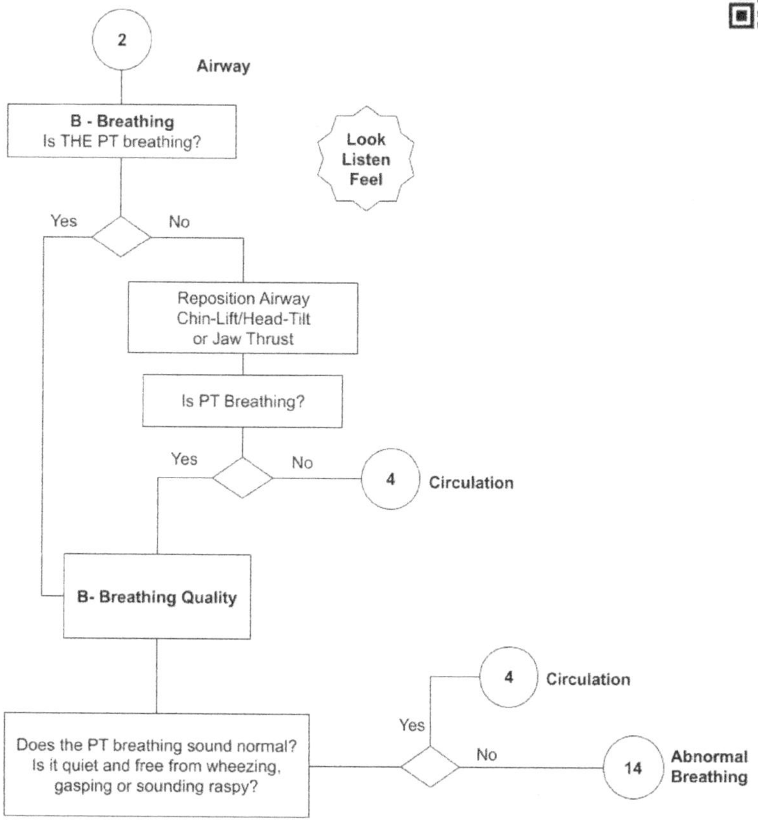

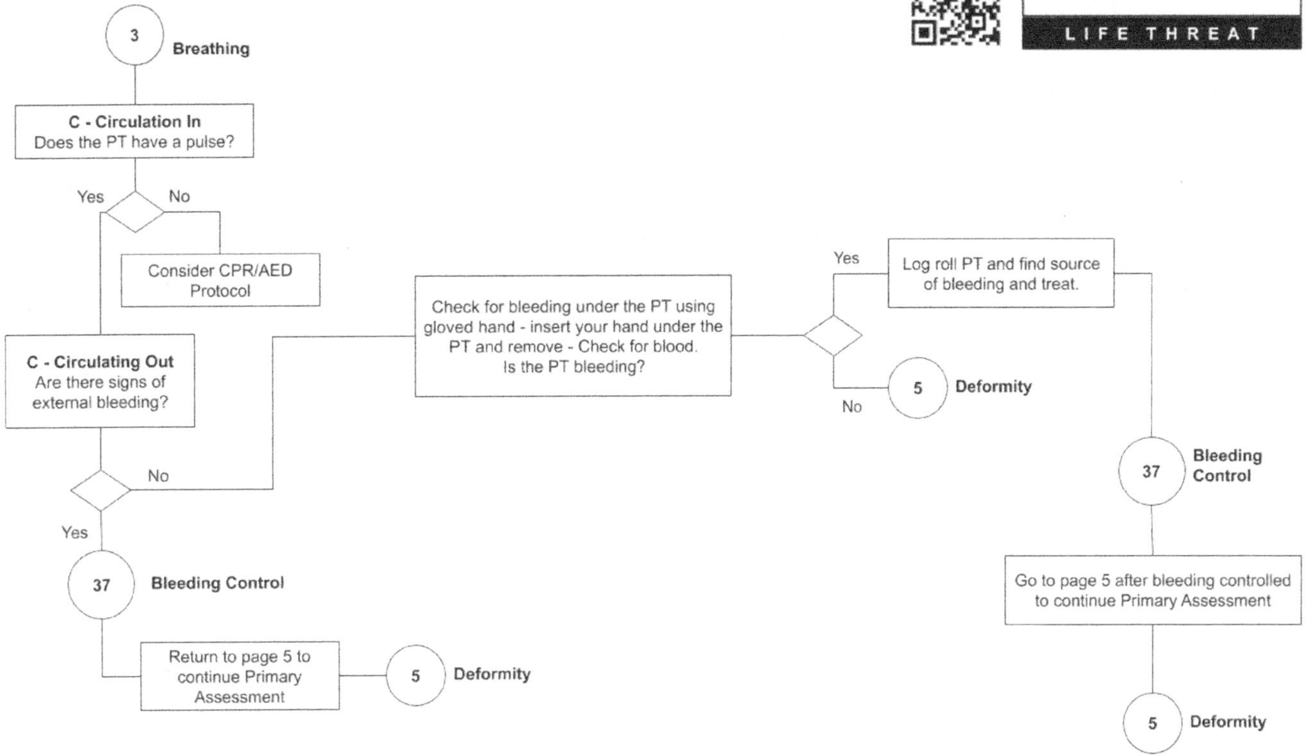
3
Breathing
C - Circulation In
Does the PT have a pulse?
Yes
No
Consider CPR/AED Protocol
C - Circulating Out
Are there signs of external bleeding?
No
Yes
37
Bleeding Control
Return to page 5 to continue Primary Assessment
5
Deformity
Check for bleeding under the PT using gloved hand - insert your hand under the PT and remove - Check for blood.
Is the PT bleeding?
Yes
Log roll PT and find source of bleeding and treat.
No
5
Deformity
37
Bleeding Control
Go to page 5 after bleeding controlled to continue Primary Assessment
5
Deformity

DEFORMITY

LIFE THREAT

5

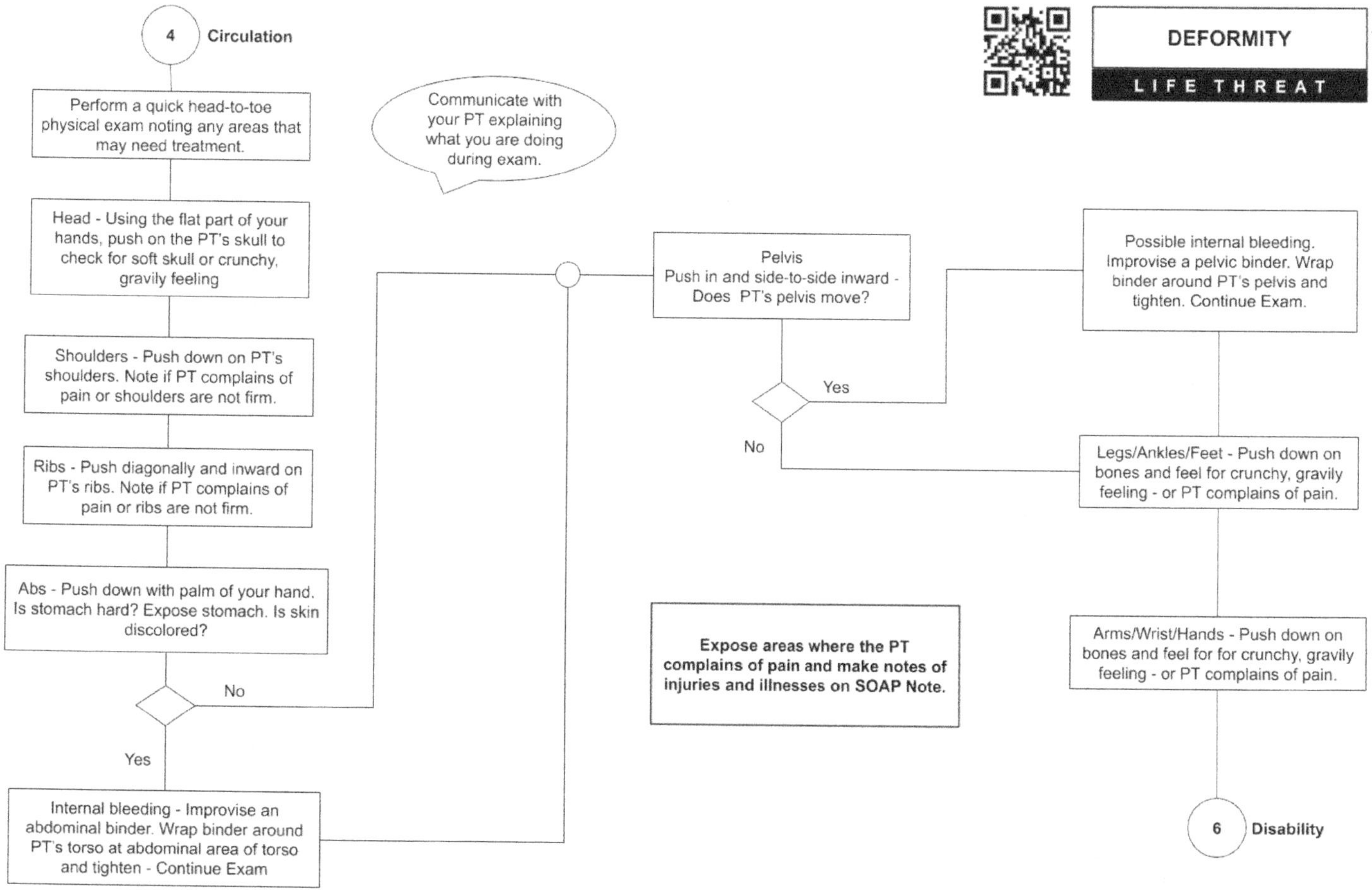

5 **Deformity**

MOVEMENT - HANDS
Place your fingers in PT's hands and ask PT to squeeze your fingers. Make note of response.

SENSATION - HANDS
Tap on one finger on each of PT's hands. Ask "What finger am I tapping?" Make note of response.

MOVEMENT - FEET
Place your hands against balls of PT's feet. Ask PT to push against your hands. Make note of response.

SENSATION - FEET
Tap on one toe on each of PT's feet. Ask "What toe am I tapping?" Make note of response.

LOG ROLL PT
-Palpate spine
-Expose and note deformities
-Expose pain points
-Look for bleeding
Is PT Bleeding?

Yes → 37 **Bleeding Control** → Return to E after bleeding controlled to continue Primary Assessment → 7 **Environment**

No → 7 **Environment**

LOG ROLL CHECKLIST

- ❑ Get a pad to protect the PT from ground.
- ❑ Place the pad of the opposite side of the PT.
- ❑ Lift PT's arm closest to the pad so that the arm is resting on the pad.
- ❑ Completely remove the reminders from the PT's head.
- ❑ Check for and remove bulky items in the PT's pocket.
- ❑ Place the PT's ankle furthest from you on top of the ankle closest to you.
- ❑ Raise PT's arms above their head. Place both arms tight up against the PT's head - no gaps between arm and head. The arm furthest from you should be on top.
- ❑ With one of your hands, grab on hips - pocket or belt loop
- ❑ With your other hand, grab high on shoulders and have your fingers touch the back of the PT's head for support.
- ❑ Roll PT toward you.
- ❑ Look for blood on PT's back side (head, back, buttocks and legs).
- ❑ Palpate entire length of spine using you hand that is holding PT's hip. Feel for vertebrae out-of-place, exposed bone or soft, crunchy bone. DO NOT remove your hand from PT's head/shoulder during exam.

Log Roll Demonstration

6 **Disability**

Roll PT onto the pad.

Protect PT from the elements heat, cold, rain, snow,

EVERYONE ELSE
Check on others in the group who may require attention.
Assign tasks to others in group.

8 **Secondary Assessment**

LOG ROLL CHECKLIST - CONTINUED

- ❑ Roll patient past 90 degrees onto your knees
- ❑ Never let go of the PT's shoulder and head
- ❑ Using the hand that was on the PT's hip, position the pad tight up against PT
- ❑ Grab PT on hip (grab a pocket or belt loop)
- ❑ Roll PT onto the pad
- ❑ Move PT's arms back down to the PT's sides
- ❑ Uncross PT's ankle and move PT's leg back to pad
- ❑ Replace reminders on PT's head

PERFORM IN ANY ORDER
Vital Signs, Physical Exam and SAMPLE History may be performed in any order.

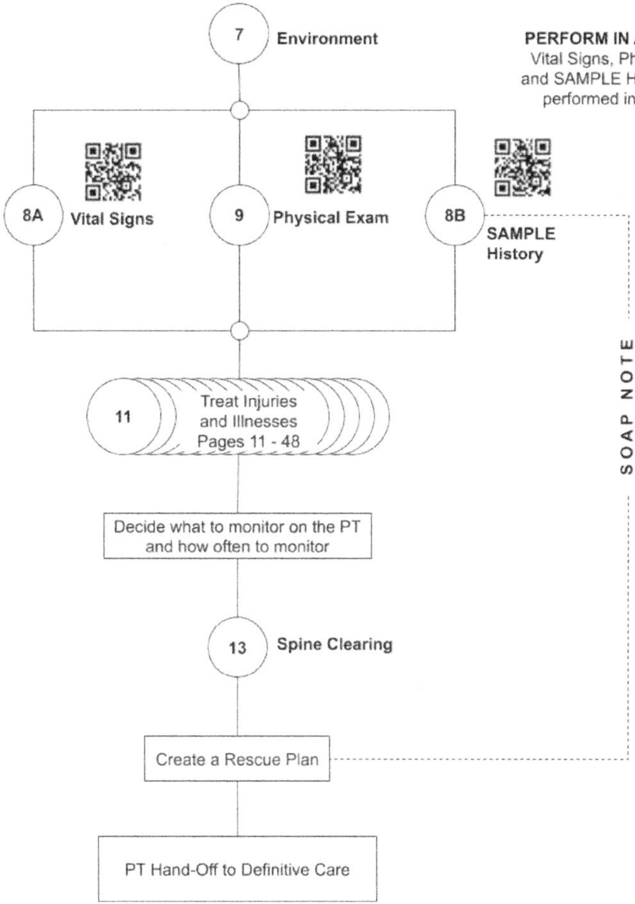

Create and Maintain a SOAP Note
Complete the SOAP Note for medical documentation and provide the SOAP Note to first responders or medical personnel at patient hand off.

VITAL SIGNS

8A

8 Secondary Assessment

Time
Record the time the PT's vitals are measured on the SOAP Note

Level of Consciousness (LOC)
Evaluate the PT's LOC by asking the PT for their name, place and time and record the results of your evaluation on the SOAP Note using the AVPU scale.

- **A**lert - Knows Name, Place & Time
  - **A+Ox3** - Correctly answers 3 of 3
  - **A+Ox2** - Correctly answers 2 of 3
  - **A+Ox1** - Correctly answers 1 of 3
  - **A Not O** - Correctly answers 0 of 3
- **V** - Verbal - PT responds to your verbal cues
- **P** - Pain - PT responds to pain
- **U** - Unresponsive - PT is unresponsive

Heart Rate
Measure and count the PT's pulse for 30 seconds. Multiply the number of heartbeats counted by 2 ard record the product on the SOAP Note.

Respiratory Rate
Observe and count number of times PT's chest rises on inhalation for 30 seconds Multiply number counted by 2 ard record the product on the SOAP Note.

Skin
Observe the PT's skin presentation and record what you see and feel on the SOAP Note.

- **Color** - Pale, Pink or Red
- **Temperature** - Cool, Hot or Warm
- **Condition** - Dry or Moist

8 Secondary Assessment

SAMPLE HISTORY

8B

(8) **Secondary Assessment**

S - Signs and Symptoms

- Signs - Record what you observe and measure on the PT
- Symptoms - Record what the PT is telling you.

A - Allergies

Ask the PT if they are allergic to anything - food, substances, insect stings and/or medications. Record the PT's response on the SOAP Note.

M - Medications

Ask the PT if they are taking any medications - prescription, over-the-counter or recreational. Record the PT's response on the SOAP Note.

P - Past Medical History

Ask about the PT's past, pertinent medical history. Record the PT's response on the SOAP Note.

L - Last In and Last Out

Ask the PT the following questions and record the responses on the SOAP Note.

- **Food - In**
  - When did they eat last?
  - What did they eat last?
  - Was the food from a trusted source?
- **Drink - In**
  - When did they drink last?
  - What did they drink last?
  - Was the drink from a trusted source?
- **Urinate - Out**
  - When did they last urinate?
  - What color was the urine
  - Did the urine have a strong smell?
- **Defecate - Out**
  - When was their last bowel movement?
  - Was it a normal bowel movement?
  - If not, how was it different?

E - Events Leading Up to the Crisis

Ask the PT about what they were doing before they began experiencing the present crisis. Record the PT's response on the SOAP Note.

(8) **Secondary Assessment**

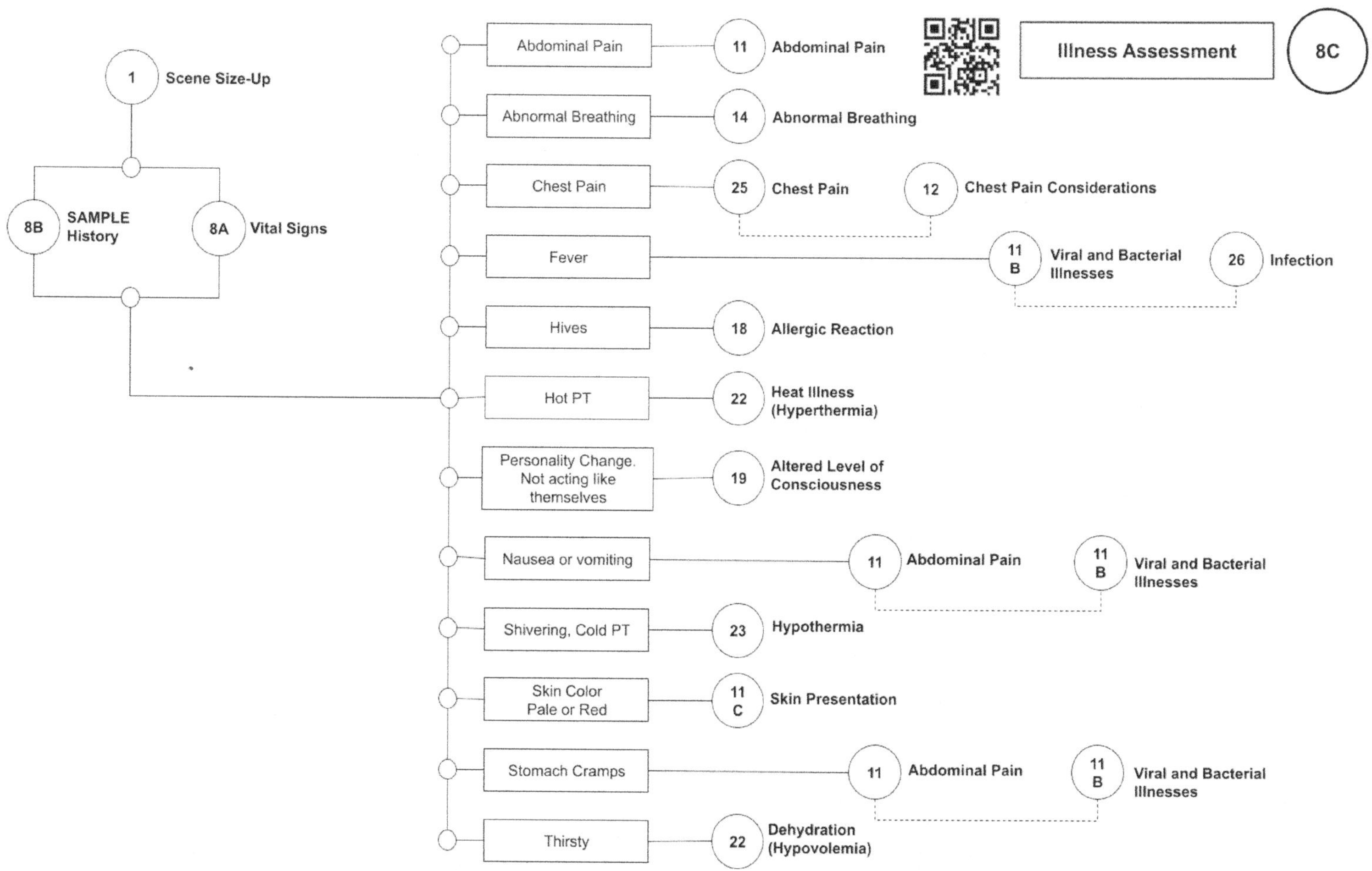

8C
Illness Assessment
1 Scene Size-Up
8B SAMPLE History
8A Vital Signs
Abdominal Pain
11 Abdominal Pain
Abnormal Breathing
14 Abnormal Breathing
Chest Pain
25 Chest Pain
12 Chest Pain Considerations
Fever
11 B Viral and Bacterial Illnesses
26 Infection
Hives
18 Allergic Reaction
Hot PT
22 Heat Illness (Hyperthermia)
Personality Change. Not acting like themselves
19 Altered Level of Consciousness
Nausea or vomiting
11 Abdominal Pain
11 B Viral and Bacterial Illnesses
Shivering, Cold PT
23 Hypothermia
Skin Color Pale or Red
11 C Skin Presentation
Stomach Cramps
11 Abdominal Pain
11 B Viral and Bacterial Illnesses
Thirsty
22 Dehydration (Hypovolemia)

SECONDARY PHYSICAL EXAM

Expose areas where the PT complains of pain and make notes of injuries and illnesses on a SOAP Note.

8 Secondary Assessment

Head
Look for signs of a
SKULL FRACTURE
-Bruising behind ears
-Bruising around eyes
-Fluid leaking from eyes, nose and ears
- Push on head using flat surfaces of the hand

FACE
Push on cheekbones, jaw bones.

NECK
- Trachea is in-line or is it pushing off to one side?
- Any blood vessels bulging?

SHOULDERS
Push on shoulder bones.
Walk fingers along collar bone

STERNUM
Push on sternum

Ribs - Push diagonally and inward.

ABDOMEN
Divide abdomen into four quadrants with the belly button in the middle of the crosshairs. Each quadrant - push in slowly and release quickly. Note - if the PT reports pain when you push in or when you release.

Pelvis
Push side-to-side and inward, Does the pelvis move?

Yes: Possible internal bleeding. Improvise a pelvic binder. Wrap binder around PT's pelvis and tighten. Continue Exam

No: Legs/Ankles/Feet - Push down on bones and feel for crunchy, gravily feeling - or PT complains of pain..

Arms/Wrist/Hands - Push down on bones and feel for for crunchy, gravily feeling - or PT complains of pain.

Joints - raise right arm, right leg, left arm, left leg. Note any limits to movement.

10 Physical Exam (Continued)

Reference - See Pages:
11 - Abdominal Pain Signs/Symptoms
12 - Chest Pain Signs/Symptoms

PHYSICAL EXAM 10

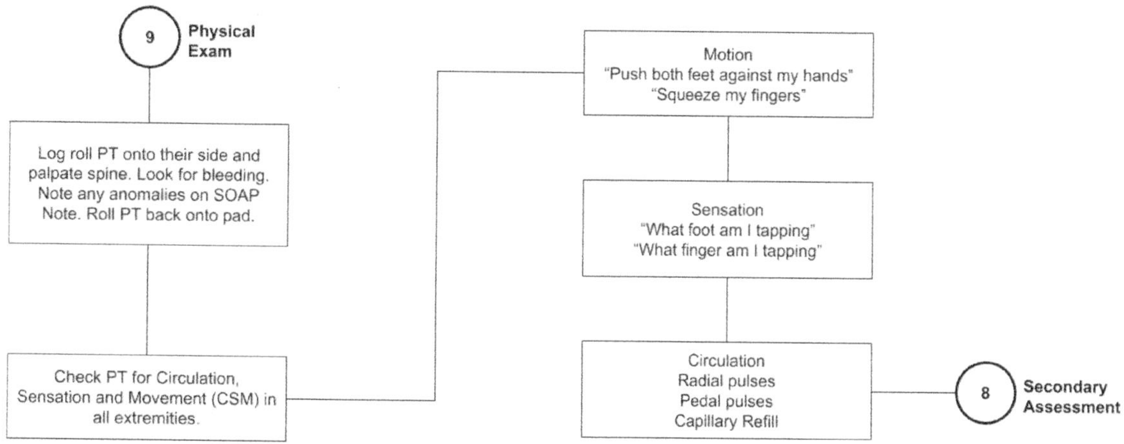

Abdominal Pain — **Perform a four-quadrant abdominal exam and refer to this table for possible illnesses**

Illness	Quadrant	Signs and Symptoms
Hernia	Anywhere	Anywhere in the abdominal area
Peritonitis	Anywhere	Anywhere in the abdominal area
Black Widow Bite	Anywhere	Rigid abdominal muscles. PT complains of severe cramps. See Page 30 - Insect Bites and Stings
Internal Bleeding	Anywhere	Distention. Abdominals hard to palpation. Skin discoloration.
Bowel Obstruction	Diffused	Crampy abdominal pain that comes and goes. Loss of appetite. Constipation. Vomiting. Inability to have a bowel movement or pass gas. Swelling of the abdomen
Gastroenteritis - "Stomach Flu" - "24-Hour Bug"	Diffused	Common cause of abdominal discomfort due to viruses, food or water contaminated by bacteria or parasites. Can be a side effect of medications. Cramping, intermittent and diffuse. May be reproducible by palpation. Sign and symptoms may include vomiting, diarrhea, malaise, fatigue, muscle aches, and low-grade fever. See Page 11B - Bacterial and Viral Illnesses.
Diverticulitis	LLQ	Left lower quadrant pain.
Kidney Stones	LLQ/RLQ	Colicky severe flank pain. Pain possibly radiating to genitalia. Maybe blood in the urine.
Ruptured ectopic pregnancy	LLQ/RLQ	Missed period, pelvic pain, abnormal vagina bleeding, dizziness
Urinary tract infection (UTI)	Lower Middle	Signs and Symptoms may include: Strong, persistent urge to urinate, burning sensation when urinating, passing frequent, small amounts of urine, possible blood in the urine, passing cloudy or strong-smelling urine, pelvic discomfort, feeling of pressure in the lower abdomen, low-grade fever
Pancreatitis	LUQ	Severe, sharp or twisting epigastric and/or LUQ pain radiating to the back.
Appendicitis	RLQ	Rebound tenderness (pain felt on rebound after palpation). Sometimes pain felt around navel (referred). Patient may complain of nausea or present in some advanced cases with vomiting, fever, shock.
Gallstones	RUQ	Acute onset of RUQ pain and tenderness. May be referred to the right shoulder. May be related to a high fat meal. Possibly nausea.
Hepatitis	RUQ	Jaundice, confusion, coma, edema, bleeding and bruising, renal failure, dehydration

See Page 11A - Abdominal Pain Evacuation Guidelines.

Suggested Evacuation Guidelines for Abdominal Pain

Evacuation for any patient who has:

- Pain inconsistent with a Urinary Tract Infection (UTI) or Gastroenteritis
- Signs and symptoms of, or the possibility of pregnancy

Evacuation for any patient with:

- Persistent or worsening gastroenteritis (crampy, diffuse, or intermittent pain) over 24 hours, spiking fever, bloody diarrhea, or dehydration
- Inability to tolerate any oral fluids more than 24 hours, especially if accompanied by diarrhea volume losses, or fever.

Rapid evacuation for a patient with abdominal pain that is:

- Persistent for 12 hours, especially if constant, localized or worsening
- Accompanied by guarding, tenderness, distension, rigidity
- Produced or aggravated by movement, jarring or walking
- Accompanied by blood in the urine, vomit, or feces
- Accompanied by fever > 102°F (39°C)
- Accompanied by signs and symptoms of shock. See Page 24 - Shock

Signs & Symptoms	Cold	Coronavirus	Flu	Food Poisoning	Gastroenteritis	Meningitis	Pneumonia	Strep Throat
Incubation Time	1 - 3 Days	2 - 14 Days	1 - 4 Days	30 minutes to 8 hours after eating tainted food	24-48 hours after exposure to virus	2 - 10 Days	12 hours to 3 Days	2 - 5 Days
Aches and Pains	NA	Often	Often	Often	Often	Often	Often - Sharp, Stabbing chest pain on inhalation	NA
Breathing Difficulty or Shortness of Breath	Rare	Often	Rare	NA	NA	Often in the form of fast breathing	Often	NA
Cough	Sometimes	Often - Dry	Often - Dry	NA	NA	Rare	Often - Productive with yellow, green mucus - sometimes bloody	NA
Diarrhea	NA	Rare	Sometimes in Children	Often and sometimes bloody	Often	Rare	Rare	NA
Fatigue	Sometimes	Often	Often	Often	Often	Often	Often	NA
Fever >100.3°F (38°C)	Rare	Often	Often	Often	Often	Often	Often	Often
Headaches	Rare	Often	Often	NA	Often	Often		NA
Loss of Taste or Smell	Rare	Often	Rare	NA	NA	Rare	Rare	NA
Rash	NA	NA	NA	NA	NA	Often - Rash that does not fade with pressure	NA	NA
Runny/Stuffy Nose	Often	NA	Rare	NA	NA	Rare	NA	NA
Sneezing	Often	Rare	Rare	NA	NA	Rare	Rare	NA
Sore Throat	Often	Sometimes	Sometimes	NA	NA	Rare	NA	Often
Stiff Neck	NA	NA	NA	NA	NA	Often	NA	NA
Stomach Cramps	NA	NA	NA	Often	Often	Rare	NA	NA
Vomiting/Nausea	NA	Sometimes	Sometimes	Often	Often and sometimes projectile vomiting	Often	Sometimes	NA
NOTES		Immediate evacuation	Evacuate	Perform SAMPLE History. Question anyone else in the group that consumed the suspected tainted food. Evacuate.	"Stomach bug" and "stomach flu" are both terms for viral gastroenteritis. Usually resolves itself in 24 hours "24 Hour Bug." Evacuate. See Page 11 to confirm.	See Page 47 Meningitis Immediate evacuation	See Page 12 Chest Pain Considerations Immediate evacuation	Red and swollen tonsils, sometimes with white patches or streaks of pus. Tiny, red spots on the roof of the mouth. Swollen lymph nodes. Immediate evacuation

SKIN PRESENTATION

11 C

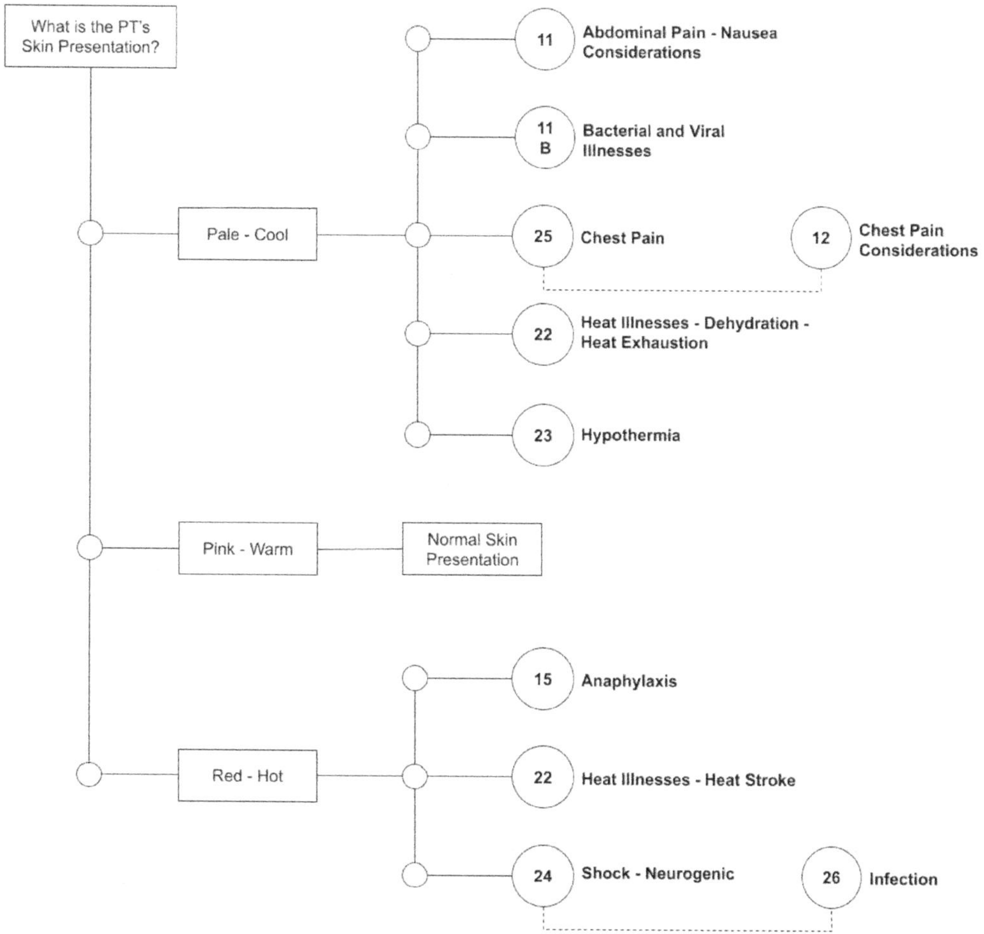

Chest Pain

Illness		Signs and Symptoms
Acute Myocardial Infarction (Heart Attack)		Chest "pressure" or epigastric pain possibly radiating to the left arm or jaw, nausea, vomiting, shortness of breath, pallor. See Page 25 Chest Pain.
Musculoskeletal		Pain on palpation, respiration. Obvious signs of trauma. Evacuate PT to the hospital.
Open Pneumothorax		Chest has been opened by a penetrating object, the hole may bubble and make a sucking noise when the patient breathes. See Page 46 Open Pneumothorax
Pleurisy		Pain on inspiration, fever, pleuritic friction rub. Evacuate PT to hospital.
Pneumonia		High fever up to 105 F. Coughing out greenish, yellow, or bloody mucus. Chills. PT feels like they can't catch their breath, especially when they move around a lot. Feeling very tired. Low appetite. Sharp or stabby chest pain when PT coughs or takes a deep breath. Sweating. Breathing and heartbeat up. Lips and fingernails turning blue. Rapid evacuation to the hospital. PT must be carried out. Do not walk PT.
Pulmonary Embolism - Blood clot in the lung		Sudden onset of shortness of breath, cough, chest pain which is sharp and pleuritic, rapid heart rate, rapid respirations, apprehension, sweating, breathing sounds: crackles.Rapid evacuation to the hospital. PT must be carried out. Do not walk PT.
Ulcer/GERD		Burning epigastric pain, nausea, vomiting, possible vomiting of blood, low blood pressure, decreased bowel sounds. Evacuate PT to the hospital.

SPINE CLEARING

13

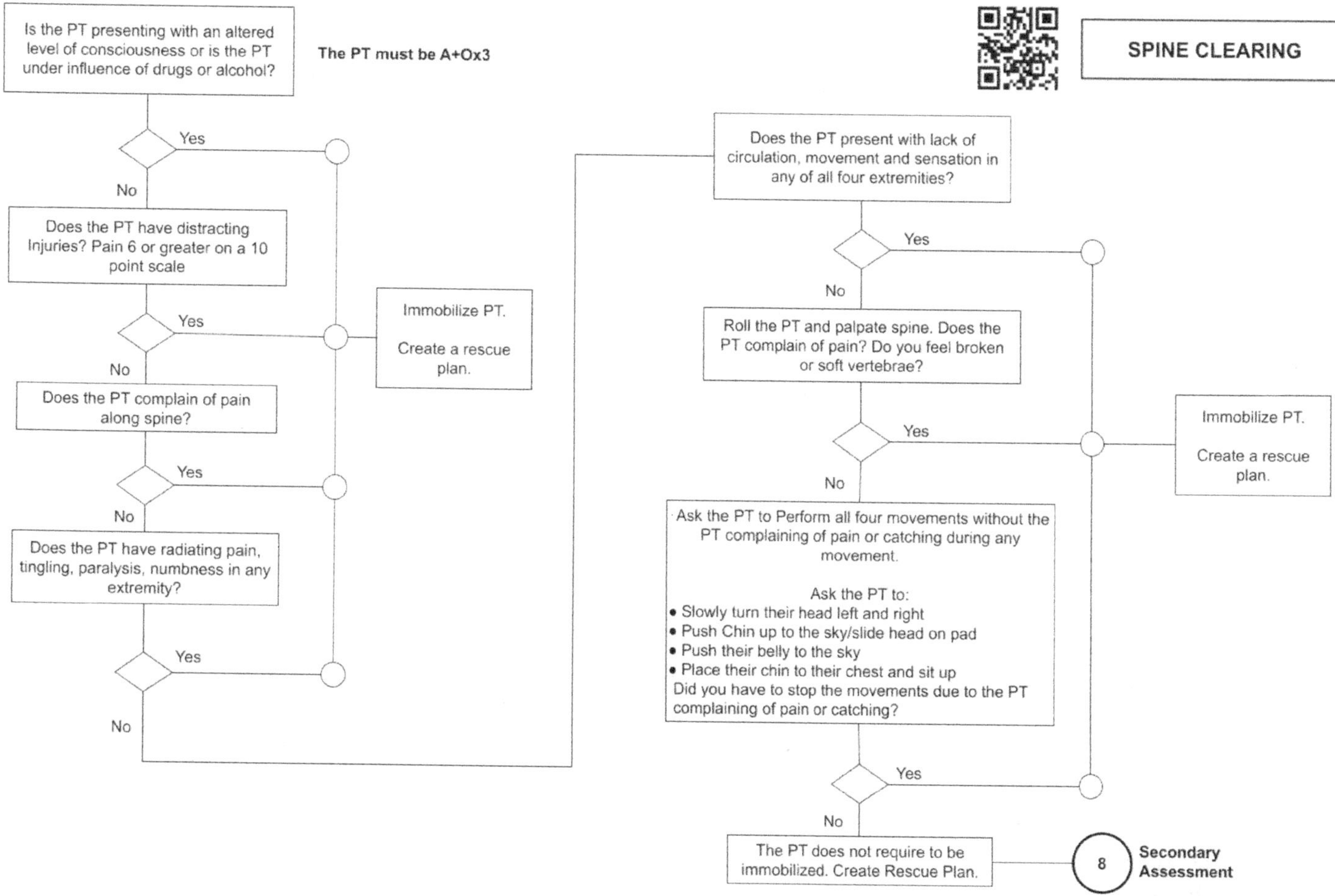

PT's breathing is not normal.

- Wheezing on Exhale → 16 Asthma
- Respiratory Distress
Swollen face, lips, tongue, airway, extremities, hives, skin color - red → 15 Anaphylaxis
- Mild to no breathing difficulty
Local swelling near a sting site.
Swelling around face, lips and extremities
Hives, Runny nose, Itchy, swollen eyes → 18 Allergic Reaction
- Shortness of breath. PT may complain of feeling ill or look ill. Possibly pale skin. → 11 B Viral and Bacterial Illnesses
- Breathing >30 Breaths/Minute
or
<6 Breaths/Minute → 17 Breathing Too Fast/Slow
- Sucking sound on inhale coming from a chest wound. → 46 Open Pneumothorax

PT CHOKING?
Perform back blows and abdominal thrusts until airway blockage is expelled.

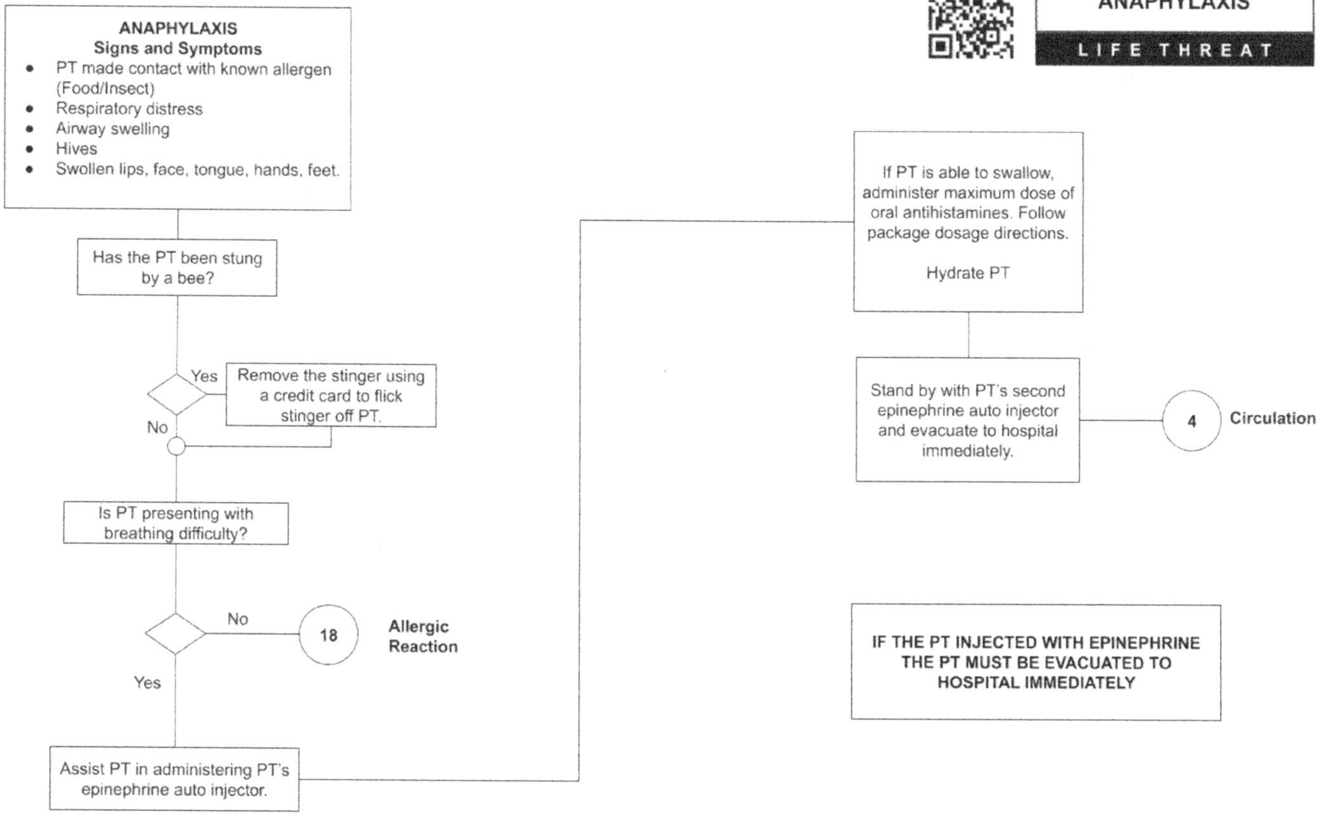
ANAPHYLAXIS
Signs and Symptoms
• PT made contact with known allergen (Food/Insect)
• Respiratory distress
• Airway swelling
• Hives
• Swollen lips, face, tongue, hands, feet.
Has the PT been stung by a bee?
Yes
Remove the stinger using a credit card to flick stinger off PT.
No
Is PT presenting with breathing difficulty?
No
18
Allergic Reaction
Yes
Assist PT in administering PT's epinephrine auto injector.
If PT is able to swallow, administer maximum dose of oral antihistamines. Follow package dosage directions.
Hydrate PT
Stand by with PT's second epinephrine auto injector and evacuate to hospital immediately.
4
Circulation
IF THE PT INJECTED WITH EPINEPHRINE THE PT MUST BE EVACUATED TO HOSPITAL IMMEDIATELY

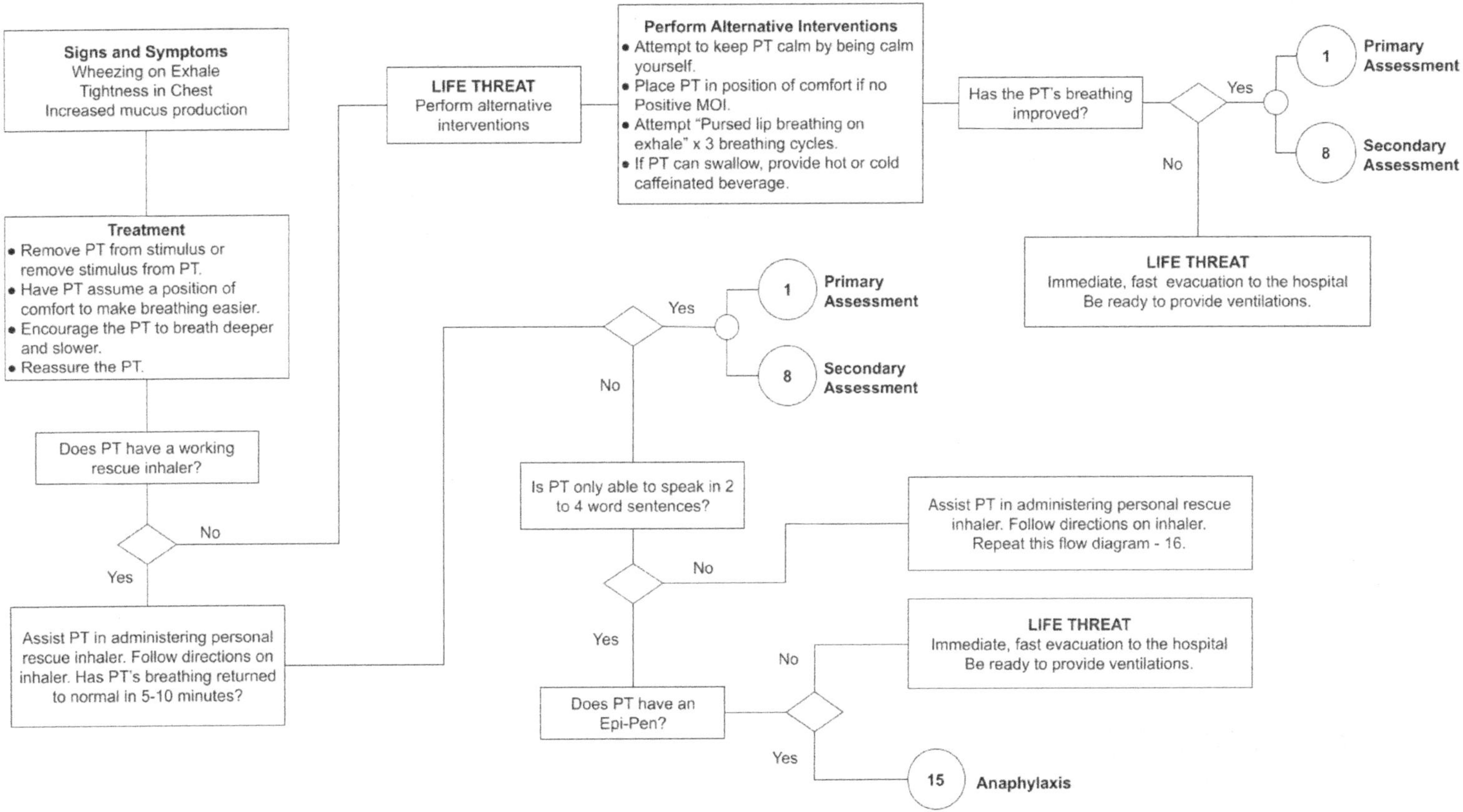
Signs and Symptoms
Wheezing on Exhale
Tightness in Chest
Increased mucus production
Treatment
• Remove PT from stimulus or remove stimulus from PT.
• Have PT assume a position of comfort to make breathing easier.
• Encourage the PT to breath deeper and slower.
• Reassure the PT.
Does PT have a working rescue inhaler?
No
Yes
Assist PT in administering personal rescue inhaler. Follow directions on inhaler. Has PT's breathing returned to normal in 5-10 minutes?
LIFE THREAT
Perform alternative interventions
Perform Alternative Interventions
• Attempt to keep PT calm by being calm yourself.
• Place PT in position of comfort if no Positive MOI.
• Attempt "Pursed lip breathing on exhale" x 3 breathing cycles.
• If PT can swallow, provide hot or cold caffeinated beverage.
Has the PT's breathing improved?
Yes
1
Primary Assessment
8
Secondary Assessment
No
LIFE THREAT
Immediate, fast evacuation to the hospital
Be ready to provide ventilations.
Yes
1
Primary Assessment
8
Secondary Assessment
No
Is PT only able to speak in 2 to 4 word sentences?
No
Assist PT in administering personal rescue inhaler. Follow directions on inhaler. Repeat this flow diagram - 16.
Yes
Does PT have an Epi-Pen?
No
LIFE THREAT
Immediate, fast evacuation to the hospital
Be ready to provide ventilations.
Yes
15
Anaphylaxis

BREATHING TOO FAST/SLOW

LIFE THREAT

17

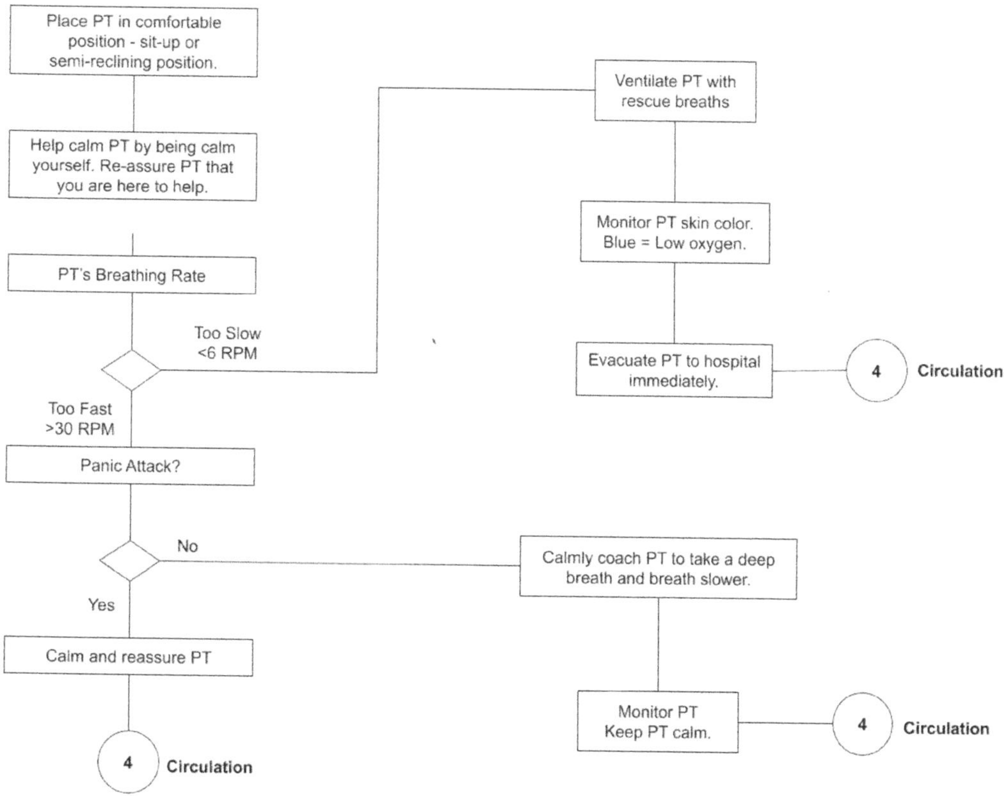

PT CHOKING?
Perform back blows and abdominal thrusts until airway blockage is expelled.

Ventilation Rates
Adults: 1 breath every 5 seconds
Children: 1 breath every 3-5 seconds

Mild to Moderate Allergic Reaction Signs and Symptoms

- PT made contact with known allergen (Food/Insect)
- Local swelling near a sting site.
- Hives
- Runny nose
- Itchy, swollen eyes
- Mild to no breathing difficulty

Has the PT been stung by a bee?

- Yes → Remove the stinger using a credit card to flick stinger off PT.
  - Is PT presenting with breathing difficulty?
    - Yes → 15 **Anaphylaxis**
    - No → Administer maximum dose of oral antihistamines.
- No → Remove allergen from the PT or remove PT from the offending environment.
  - Is PT presenting with breathing difficulty?
    - Yes → 15 **Anaphylaxis**
    - No → Administer maximum dose of oral antihistamines.

Administer maximum dose of oral antihistamines. Follow package dosage Hydrate PT

Monitor PT for 30+ minutes. Monitor breathing.

Is PT presenting with breathing difficulty?

- Yes → 15 **Anaphylaxis**
- No → 4 **Circulation**

Evacuation Guidelines

No History of Anaphylaxis

If the patient does not have a history of anaphylaxis, a mild to moderate allergic reactions can be treated in the field and do not require evacuation.

Priory History of Anaphylaxis

For a patient with a history of anaphylaxis to a known allergen who has been treated with an oral antihistamine, the patient should be evacuated to definitive care for evaluation. The patient may experience rapid onset of anaphylaxis when the oral antihistamine wears off in 3 to 4 hours.

19 ALTERED LEVEL OF CONSCIOUSNESS

Signs and Symptoms

- Disoriented
- Dizzy
- May be thirsty and/or hungry
- Altered Level of Consciousness
- PT not acting like themselves

Treatment

Sugar PT is not too hot, too cold, breathing is normal, not suffered a blow to their head.	**21**	Low Blood Sugar (Hypoglycemia)
Temperature PT too hot?	**22**	Heat Injuries (Hyperthermia)
Temperature PT too cold?	**23**	Cold Injuries (Hypothermia)
Oxygen Is PT presenting shortness of breath?	**14**	Abnormal Breathing
Pressure Has PT experienced a blow to their head?	**20**	Brain Injuries
Pressure Has the PT ascended to a higher altitude?	**34**	Altitude Sickness
Facial Droop, Muscle Weakness, Slurred Speech	**48**	Stroke
Drugs, Electrolytes, Electrocution, Poisons	**1**	Primary Assessment

PT has suffered blow to the head. Did PT lose consciousness - even for just a minute or so?

Yes: Evacuate PT to hospital

No or Don't Know: Are there obvious signs of head trauma, skull fracture or decrease in level of consciousness?

Yes: Immediate, Fast Evacuation to the hospital

No:

Signs and Symptoms
(One or many within 24 hours of injury)

- Abnormal speech
- Any new sensitivities to include, headache, sensitivity to noise or light
- Memory issues
- Altered Level of Consciousness - A+O<3
- Irregular breathing or hyperventilation
- Vomiting
- Bruising around eyes or behind ear(s).
- White fluid leaking from eyes, nose and/or ears,
- Heart rate decreasing
- Systolic blood pressure increasing
- Loss of motor skills
- Pupils not PERRL
- Decorticate or Decerebrate posturing (Late sign)

Does PT present with one or more of these signs and symptoms within 24 hours?

Yes:

Evacuation to Hospital

- Rapid, fast evacuation to hospital
- Maintain airway
- Control scalp bleeding
- Do not prevent draining of CSF fluid.
- Place PT in horizontal position on a backboard. Elevate the head of the backboard 30 - 40 degrees to reduce pressure in the PT's brain
- Keep PT warm
- Keep PT calm

No: PT is not presenting with the signs and symptoms of a brain injury.

HYPOGLYCEMIA
LOW BLOOD SUGAR

Signs and Symptoms
- Altered Level of Consciousness
- Change in personality
- Cranky, unhappy
- PT not acting like their normal self

Treatment
- Run SAMPLE History. Ask PT, " When is the last time you ate something?" "What did you eat?"
- Administer 15 grams of sugar (approx 1 heaping tablespoon) to PT.
- Responsive PT - Sugar can be delivered by pouring into gums and dissolving or dissolved in liquid and consumed
- Unresponsive PT - Place PT in Recovery Position - rub 15 grams of sugar into PT's gums
- Wait 10 - 15 minutes and re-evaluate PT's LOC

PT's LOC improved?

Yes → 8 Secondary Assessment

No → 19 Altered Level of Consciousness

Dehydration

Signs and Symptoms
- Thirst
- Headache
- Urine - dark, pungent
- Heat cramps -possibly
- Dehydration - Blood volume down - can lead to Hypovolemic Shock
- Dehydration untreated leads to HEAT EXHAUSTION

Treatment
- Hydrate and electrolytics
- Water with salt
- Pedialyte powder, electrolyte powder
- Melons
- Sports drinks - dilute 20% sports drink and 80% water
- Monitor PT for 30 minutes

Heat Exhaustion

Signs and Symptoms
- Dehydration S/S - Lethargic, nausea, dizzy, fatigue, mild headache
- Blood Volume DOWN - Dehydrated - Hypovolemic
- Respiratory Rate - Up a little
- Heart Rate - Up a little
- Skin - Pale, Cool, Moist
- Brain still not getting enough oxygen so PT is lethargic, dizzy and fatigued
- Heat exhaustion untreated leads to HEAT STROKE - LIFE THREAT

Heat Stroke
LIFE THREAT

Signs and Symptoms
- Skin - Red and hot.
- Vomiting
- Respiratory Rate - Way up
- Heart Rate - Way up
- LOC - Disoriented heavily, confused, personality change, combative, hallucinating, maybe unconscious, eventually coma and death
- Body temp - 105 F+,

Treatment
- Remove PT from heat - Remove excess clothing
- Hydrate PT with electrolytes - See Dehydration Treatment
- Apply cool, moist compresses to PT's neck, armpits and groin -Cool with flowing water
- Fan PT vigorously - If PT shivers - stop fanning
- Massage limbs vigorously
- Evacuation
  - Heat Exhaustion - If PT does not fully recover, evacuate to hospital
  - Heat Stroke - **LIFE THREAT** - Fast evacuation to hospital

8 Secondary Assessment

HYPOTHERMIA

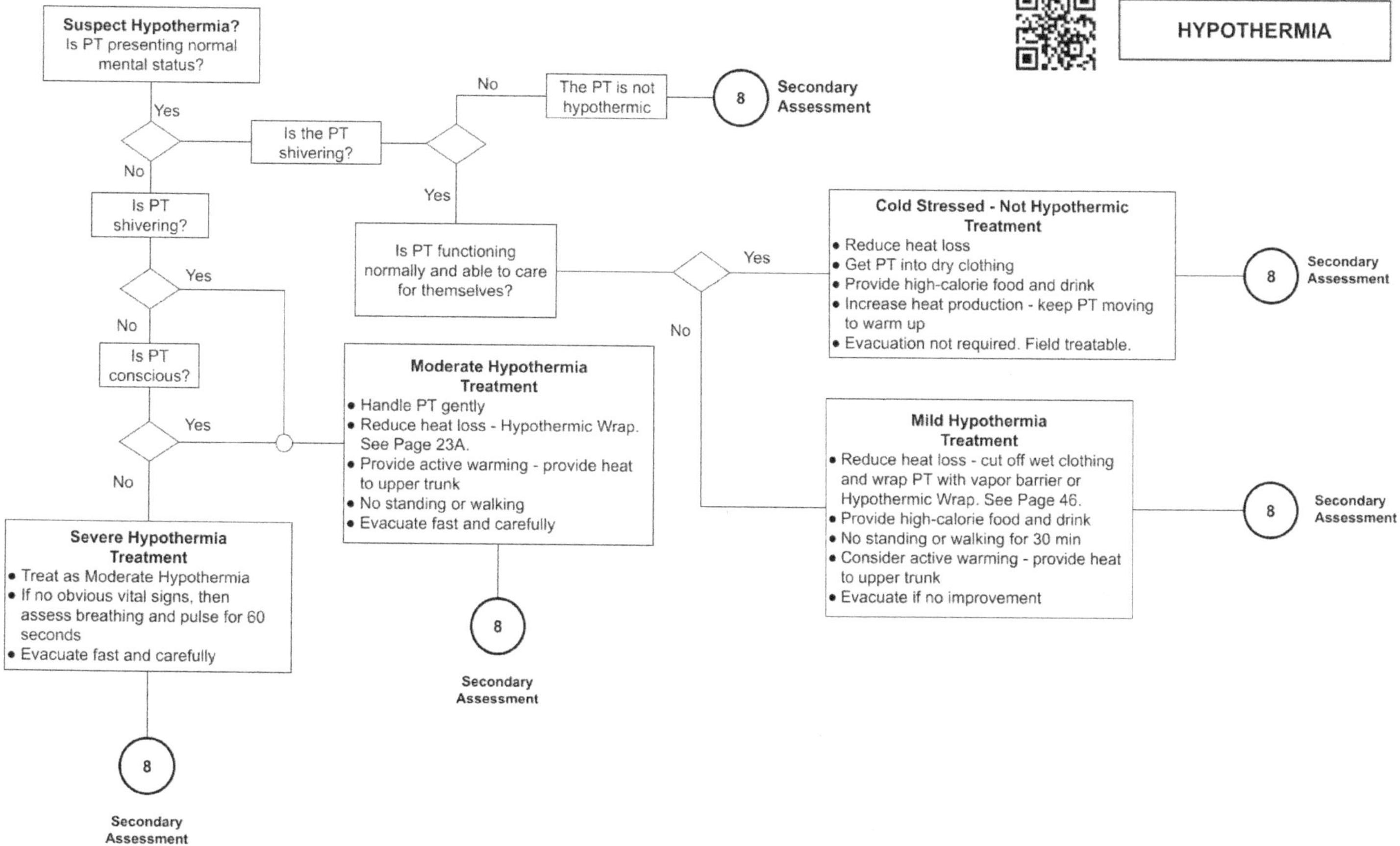

Component List

- Large tarp or plastic sheeting
- Foam pad(s)
- Sleeping bag, blankets, quilts, etc. If using sleeping bag, place patient in bag and zip up completely.
- Internal vapor barrier - tarp or plastic sheeting - required if patient's clothes are damp or wet - see Instructions
- Active rewarming heat source - warm water bottles/bladder.

Instructions

Dry Clothing - Leave clothes on patient. Internal vapor barrier optional.

Damp Clothing - Leave clothing on and use internal vapor barrier against to keep sleeping bag/blankets from getting wet.

Wet Clothing
Definitive care less than 30 minutes away - Wrap patient immediately and transport.

Definitive care more than 30 minutes away - Protect the patient from getting colder, remove wet clothing and wrap.

Active Rewarming
If heat is placed in patient armpits and chest - ensure layer of material between patient and heat source. Monitor patient's skin for redness due to too warm heat source.

1

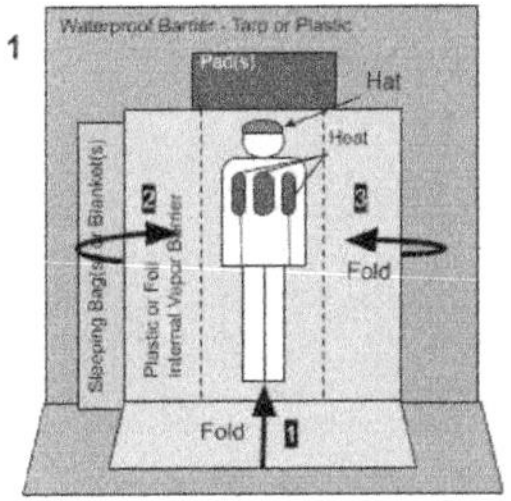

2

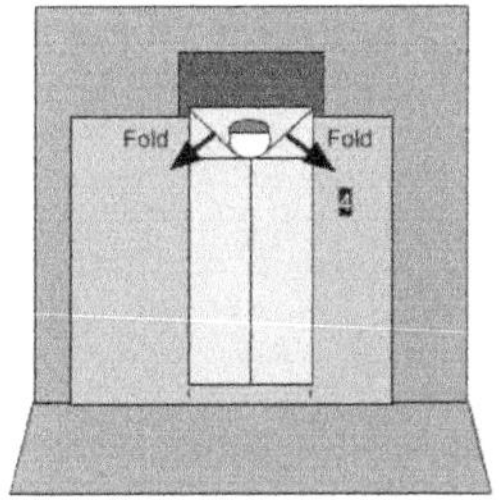

3

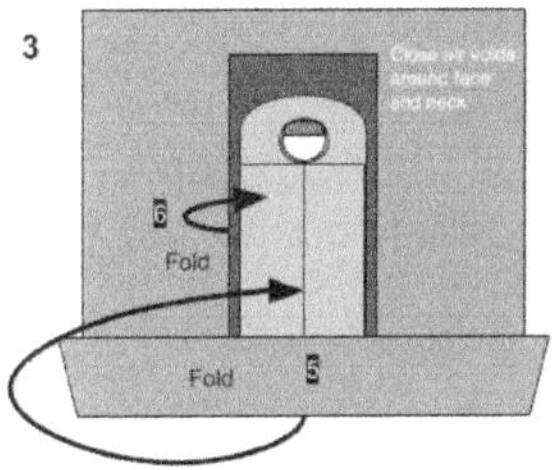

4

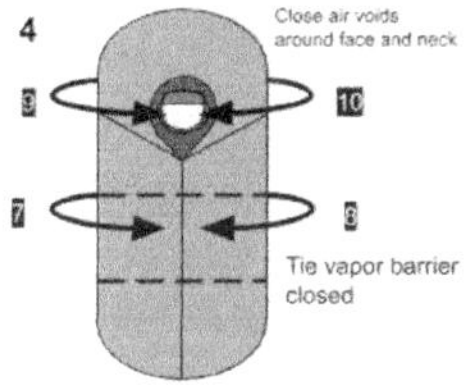

TYPE	CAUSE	VASCULAR RESPONSE	SKIN
Cardiogenic	Heart Problem	Vasoconstrict	Pale, cool
Hypovolemic	Bleed Out/In Severe Dehydration	Vasoconstrict	Pale, cool
Neurogenic (Distributive)	• Septic • Anaphylaxis • Spinal Cord Injury	Vasodilation	Red, hot, moist or dry

25 Chest Pain

4 Circulation

22 Dehydration Heat Illnesses

15 Anaphylaxis

26 Infection

Signs and Symptoms

- LOC : Falling. Not acting like themselves. Disoriented
- RR : Rising, shallow
- HR: Rising, weak
- SKIN: See "Skin" column
- Blood Pressure: Falling

Treatment

- Lay down, keep warm
- If PT can swallow, give PT small and frequent sips of water
- Treat problem causing shock
  See pages 4, 15, 22, 25 and 26
- Evacuate to hospital

Guidelines for Evacuation

Evacuate any patient with signs and symptoms of shock that do not stabilize or improve over time.

Evacuate rapidly any patient with decreased mental status or worsening vital signs. All patients presenting with shock will need to be carried.

Cardiac S/S - One or More

- Chest pain - tightness, pressure, possibly radiating into arm and/or neck/jaw
- Upper abdominal pain
- Weakness
- Nausea
- Denial
- Shock
- Sweating
- Anxious
- Sense of impending doom
- FEMALE PT - "Bra feels tight"

Treatment

Place PT in position of rest and comfort. Sitting or reclining.

Keep PT and others calm. If PT asks if they are having a heart attack your answer is "I don't know, but I am going to take good care of you and stay with you until EMS arrives."

Ask SAMPLE history.

If PT is not allergic to aspirin then administer 4 chewable aspirin (4 x 81 mg) or 1 regular aspirin.

Allow PT to take small, frequent sips of water to hydrate them.

If PT is prescribed nitroglycerin then assist PT in taking medicine. DO NOT TOUCH NITROGLYCERIN PILL.

Calmly evacuate PT to hospital.

8 **Secondary Assessment**

See Page 12 for other chest pain considerations

INFECTION

LOCAL INFECTION
Signs/Symptoms
- Swelling
- Hot
- Ache
- Red
- Pus

Treatment
Clean area around infected area with soap and water

Sterilize safety pin - poke holes and drain pus.

Clean area area with soap and water.

Soak infected area in hot, salty water or moist, salty heat pack or apply honey to affected area.

Apply sterile bandage, Monitor infected area every few hours to check for infection.

8 Secondary Assessment

SYSTEMIC INFECTION
LIFE THREAT!
Signs/Symptoms
- Local infected area with a red streak radiating and moving toward heart.
- Swollen lymph nodes
- Fever and/or chills
- Septic shock

Treatment
Treat local infected area.

Clean area around infected area with soap and water

Sterilize safety pin - poke holes and drain pus.

Clean area area with soap and water.

Soak infected area in hot, salty water or moist, salty heat pack or apply honey to affected area.

Apply sterile bandage, Monitor infected area every few hours to check for infection.

If infected area located on an extremity - immobilize extremity below the heart.

Evacuate PT to hospital.

8 Secondary Assessment

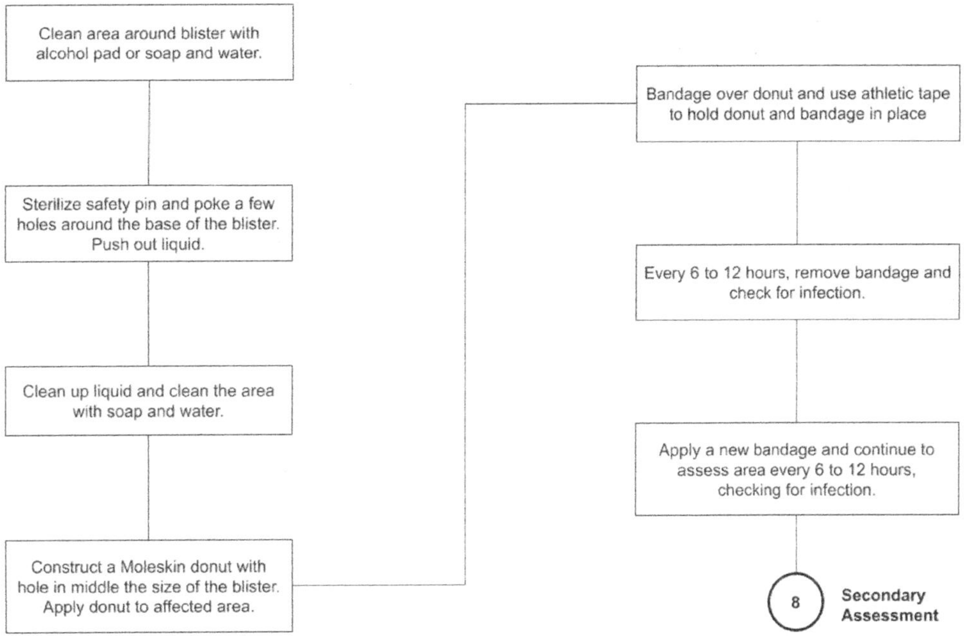
Clean area around blister with alcohol pad or soap and water.
Sterilize safety pin and poke a few holes around the base of the blister. Push out liquid.
Clean up liquid and clean the area with soap and water.
Construct a Moleskin donut with hole in middle the size of the blister. Apply donut to affected area.
Bandage over donut and use athletic tape to hold donut and bandage in place
Every 6 to 12 hours, remove bandage and check for infection.
Apply a new bandage and continue to assess area every 6 to 12 hours, checking for infection.
8
Secondary Assessment

FRACTURES, SPRAINS AND STRAINS

28

Signs and Symptoms
Fractures, Sprains and Strains

- Guarding
- Swelling
- Discoloration
- Warm
- Pain
- Bear Weight
- Movement

Palpate injured area. What type of pain does the PT complain of?

General soreness

Sprain or Strain

Treatment
Sprain and Strains

- Rest
- Ice
- Compression
- Elevate

8

Secondary Assessment

Sharp point pain

Fracture
Signs and Symptoms

May include one or more of the following:

- Crepitus
- Agulation
- Open fracture
- Decreased distal circulation, sensation and movement (CSM)

Treatment
Fractures

- Remove jewelry from injured extremity
- Remove shoe if leg fracture
- Rest
- Ice
- Compression
- Elevate (after splinting)
- Check circulation, sensation and movement (CSM)
- If CSM absent - traction-in-line extremity to set fracture and restore CSM

28 A

Arm Splinting

28 D

Leg Splinting

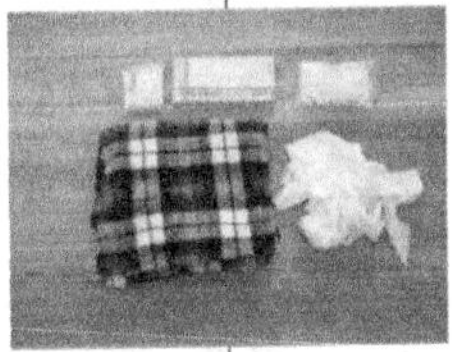

Arm Splint Supply List

1 - SAM Splint or Rigid Elements
1 - Padded Material
7 - Cloth strips, each 18 - 24" long
1 - Cloth strip long enough to wrap around PT's torso and slung arm
1 - Triangle bandage
1 - Cool pack

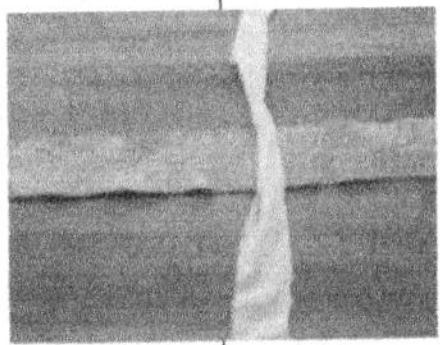

Remove the SAM Splint from its packaging and unfold it completely. Near the middle of the unfolded SAM Splint we will take a strip that is approximately 2 feet long and lay it exactly in the middle of the SAM Splint.

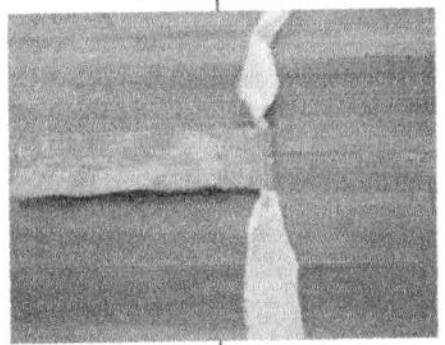

Fold the SAM Splint once over the strip.

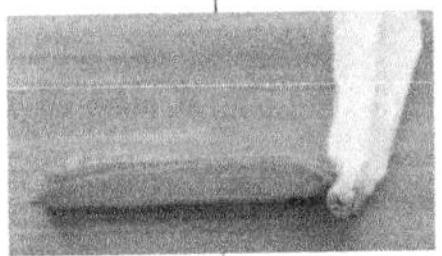

Roll the SAM Splint at the strip a few times. This will be where the Patient's hand will rest, and we can adjust the length of the SAM Splint by the number of times we roll the splint.

ARM SPLINTING

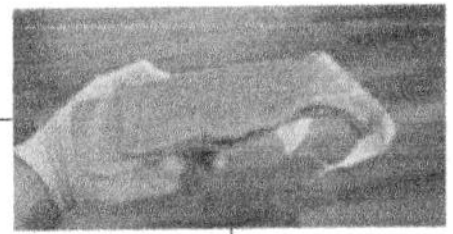

Bend the remainder of the SAM Splint into a "V". This V-bend will make the SAM Splint rigid.

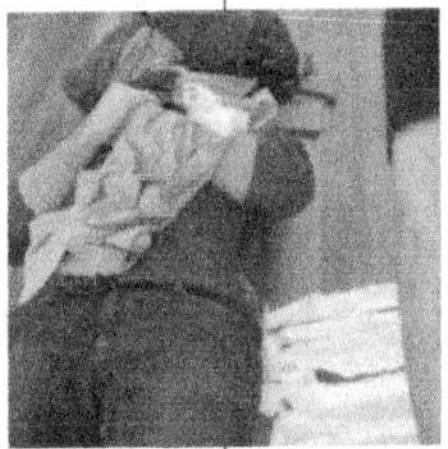

We will build the splint next to the patient, who will be laying on a pad on the ground. We will first lay our strips of cloth on the ground next to our patient.

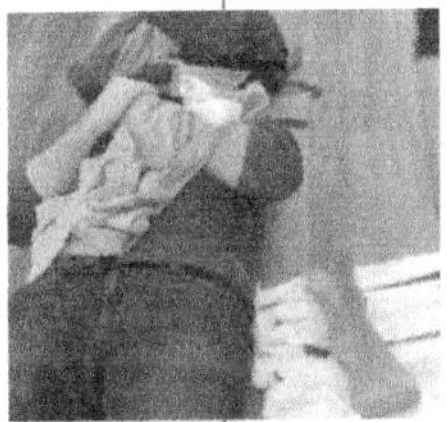

Lay the prepared SAM Splint on top of the strips of cloth.

28 B Arm Splinting

ARM SPLINTING

28 B

28 A Arm Splinting

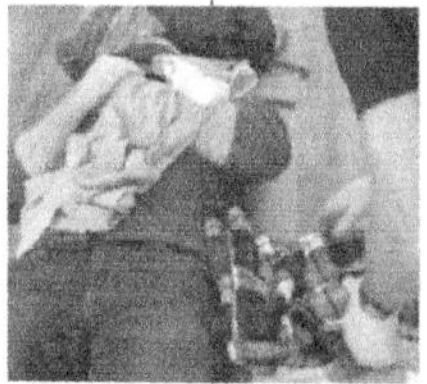

Lay the padding material on top of the prepared SAM Splint.

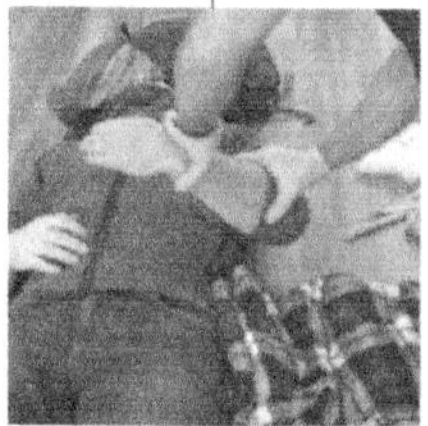

Check patient again for jewelry. Remove jewelry from patient's injured extremity. Using both hands, gently lift and move the patient's arm into the splint.

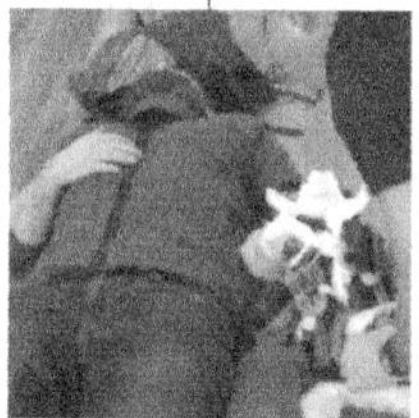

Tie the splint closed. Do not tie directly over the injury. Leave an open area in the padding above the injured area to insert a cool pack.

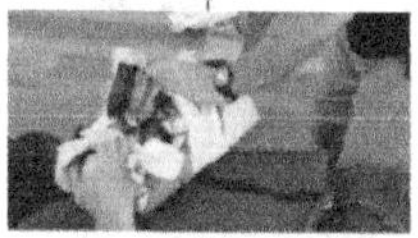

Move the patient's arm to their chest. Check for circulation, sensation and movement every 15 minutes.

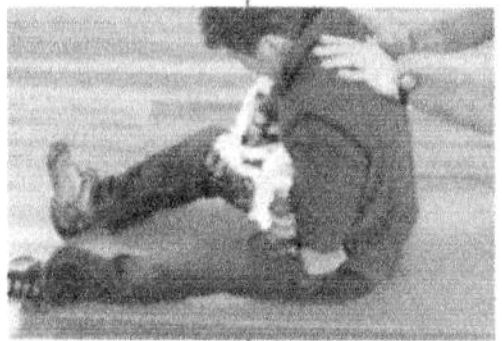

Clear the PT's spine using the Spine Clearing Flow Diagram found on Page 13. If you are able to successfully clear the patient's spine, then you can sit and stand the patient. If you cannot clear the patient's spine, then secure the patient's arm to their chest and immobilize the patient.

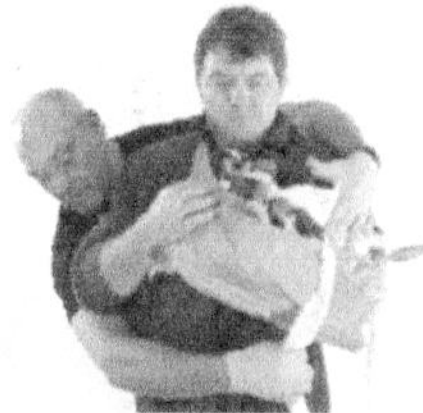

Tie a knot in one end of a triangle bandage. This will create a pocket for the patient's elbow to rest. Tie the other two corners of the triangle bandage behind the patient's neck and this will create a sling. Tie the sling so the patient's hand is in an elevated position.

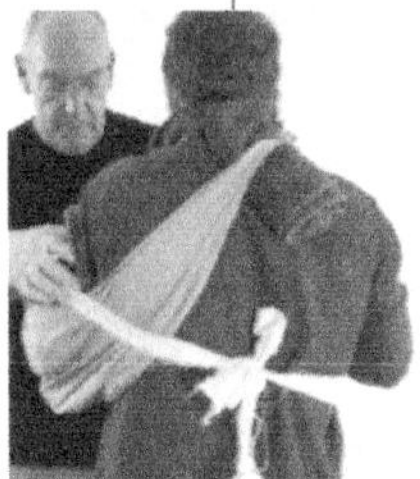

Tie a cloth strip across the patient's elbow, around the patient's torso and tie the strip at the patient's back. This is to secure the patient's elbow to the patient's torso, reducing excess movement of the splinted arm. Create a pad using fabric, foam or other soft material. Place this pad between the patient's neck and the sling for patient comfort.

28 C Arm Splinting

Arm Splint Quality Checklist

- ☐ Six (6) cloth strips - tightly tied. Not able to slide a finger between strips and SAM splint.
- ☐ Pad placed between patient's neck and sling.
- ☐ Padded material encircles arm 360 degrees. Injury area assessable for cool pack.
- ☐ Arm slightly elevated.
- ☐ Strip tied to secure hand to splint. Strip runs between thumb and forefinger.
- ☐ Natural curl of fingers over rolled splint. Fingers are accessible to test circulation, sensation and movement (CSM).
- ☐ All jewelry removed from fingers, hand and arm.
- ☐ SAM Splint - Rolled for hand and "V"-bent for rigidity.

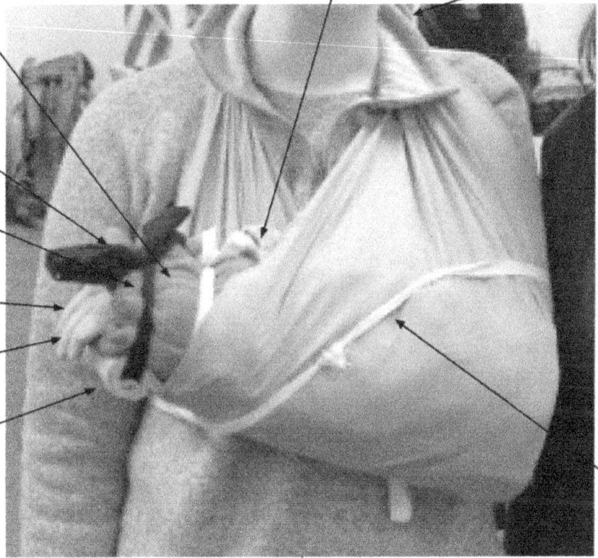

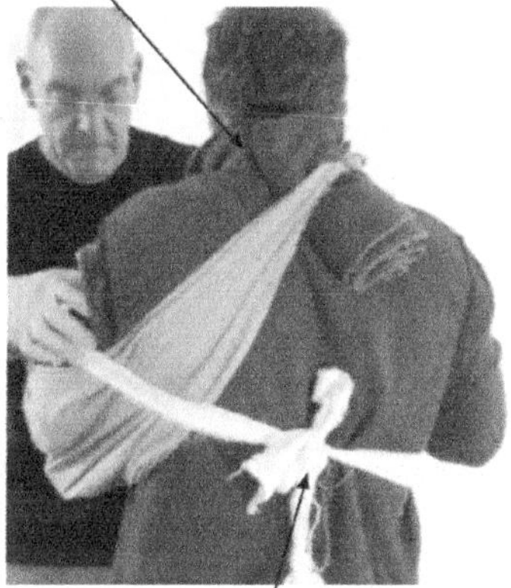

- ☐ Arm secured to patient's torso using a cloth strip.

8
Secondary Assessment

28 Fractures, Sprains and Strains

LEG SPLINTING

28 D

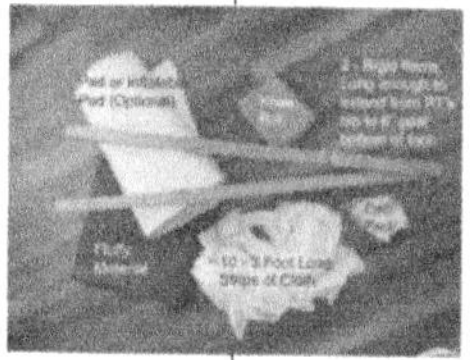

Leg Splint Supply List

2 - Rigid Elements
1 - Padded Material
12 - Cloth strips, each at least 24" long
1 - Cloth roll for behind knee
1 - Optional foam or inflatable pad
1 - Cool pack

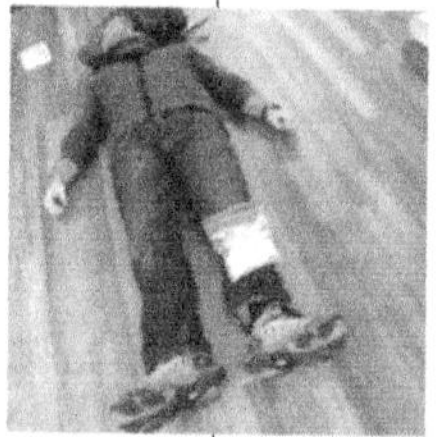

Place cool pack on injured area. If you are using an ice pack, place material between ice pack and patient's skin

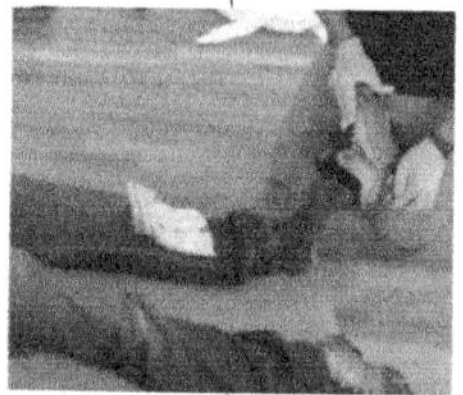

Remove the patient's footware.

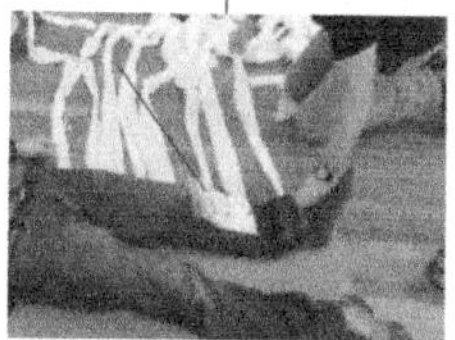

Build splint next to the patient. Lay down eight cloth strips - four above the knee - four below the knee.

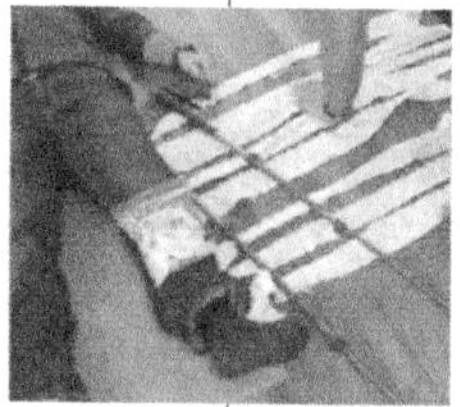

Lay the rigid elements on top of the cloth strips. Anticipate where the patient's leg will lay when you move it into the splint.

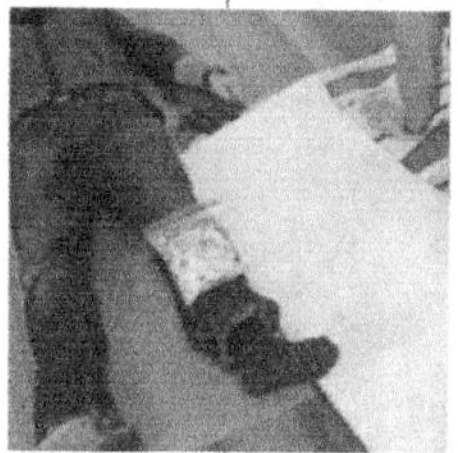

If you have an optional pad, lay the pad on top of the rigid elements. You may fold the pad so that it extends 12" past the patient's foot, or you may roll the pad to the patient's foot once the splint is tied closed..

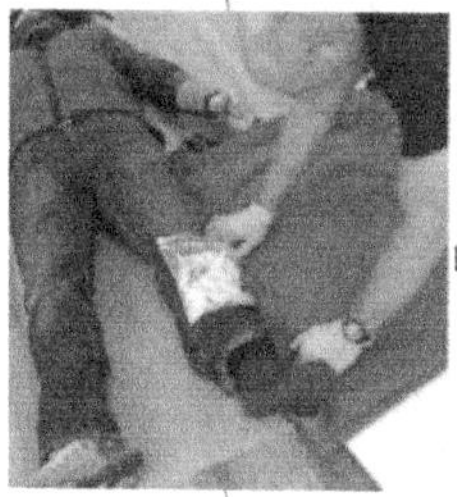

Lay the padded material in place.

28E Leg Splinting

28D Leg Splinting

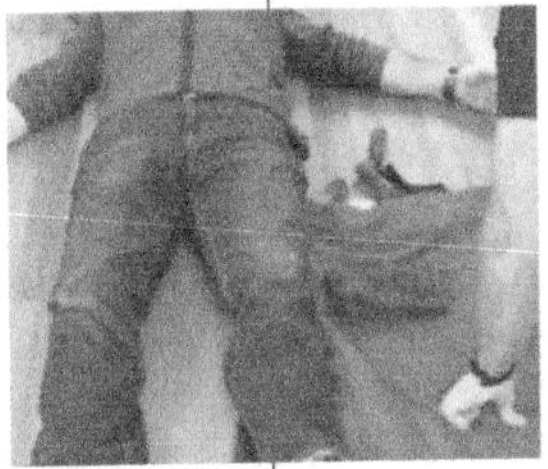

Roll up cloth and place on padded material where the back of the patient's knee will land when the leg is moved into the splint.

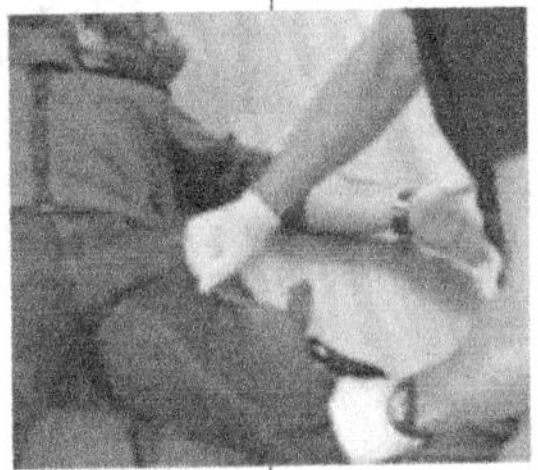

Using two hands, move the patient's leg into the splint.

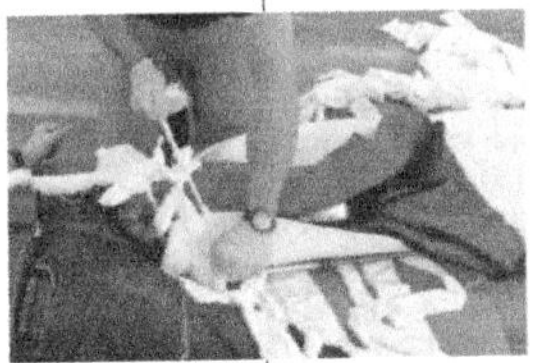

Tie the splint closed with the eight strips of cloth.

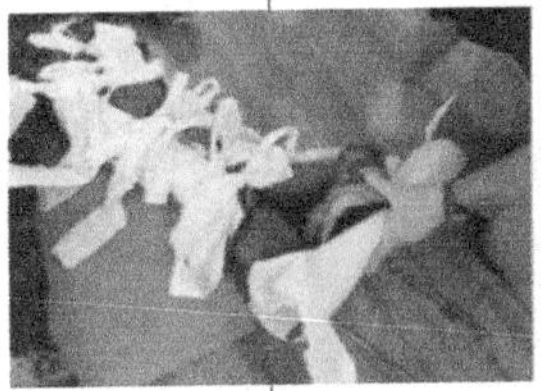

Optional pad - If you did not bend the pad back, roll pad against patient's foot. Insert patient's footwear between patient's sole of foot and splint.

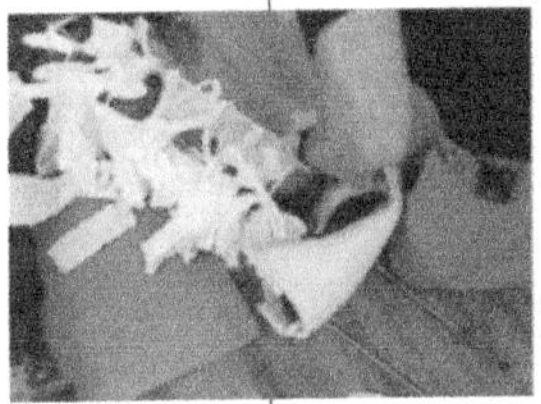

Tie the splint so the patient can not push with their foot.

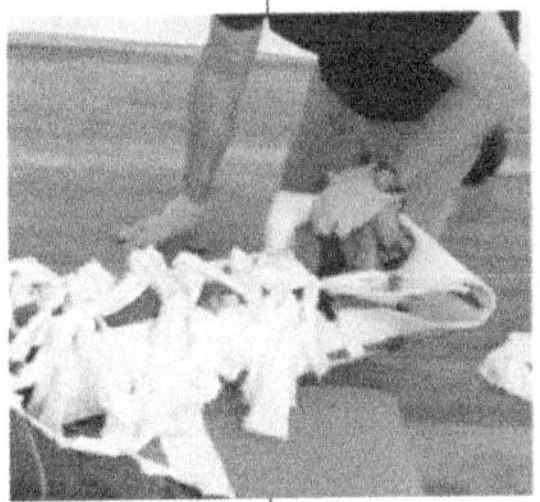

Tie the splint so the patient can not move their foot backwards.

28F Leg Splinting

28
F

LEG SPLINTING

Leg Splint Quality Checklist

- ❑ Two rigid elements
- ❑ Rigid elements extend from patient's crotch and hip to at least six inches past the patient's foot.
- ❑ Eight adjustable strips - four above the knee and four below the knee
- ❑ Padded material encircles the leg 360 degrees
- ❑ Small roll of fabric or foam is placed behind patient's knee
- ❑ Strips are tight. Not able to insert a finger between strips and rigid elements
- ❑ Patient's leg is immobilized. Patient cannot bend their knee
- ❑ Patient's footwear is removed on injured leg
- ❑ Patient's foot is immobilized - patient cannot move their foot
- ❑ Caregiver has access to patient's toes to check for circulation, sensation and movement
- ❑ Caregiver has access to injury area to place a cool pack

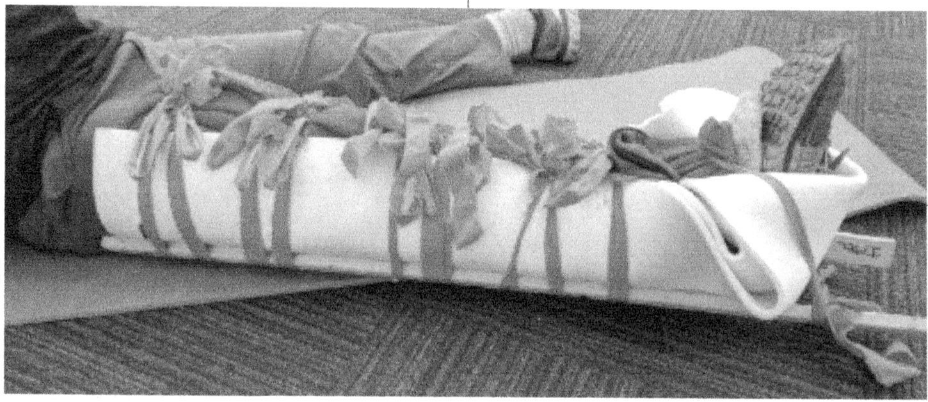

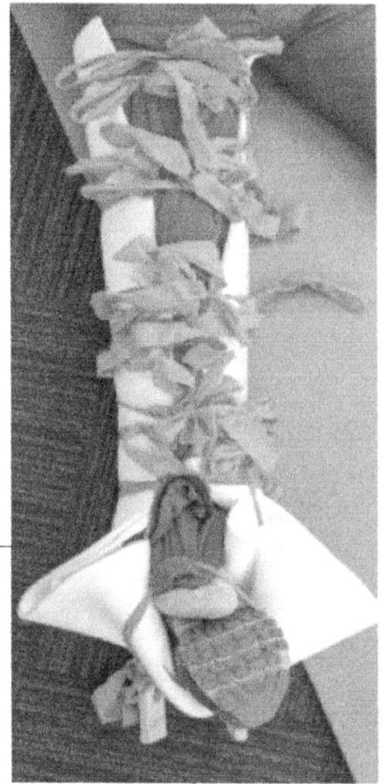

9 Secondary Assessment

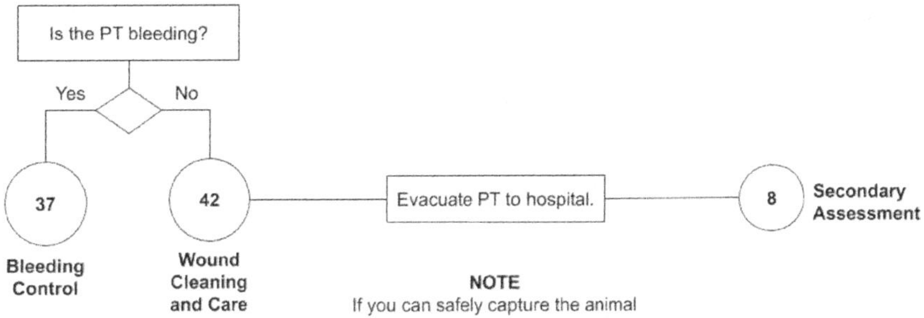

NOTE

If you can safely capture the animal dead or alive - transport animal to Health Department for testing.

30 INSECT BITES AND STINGS

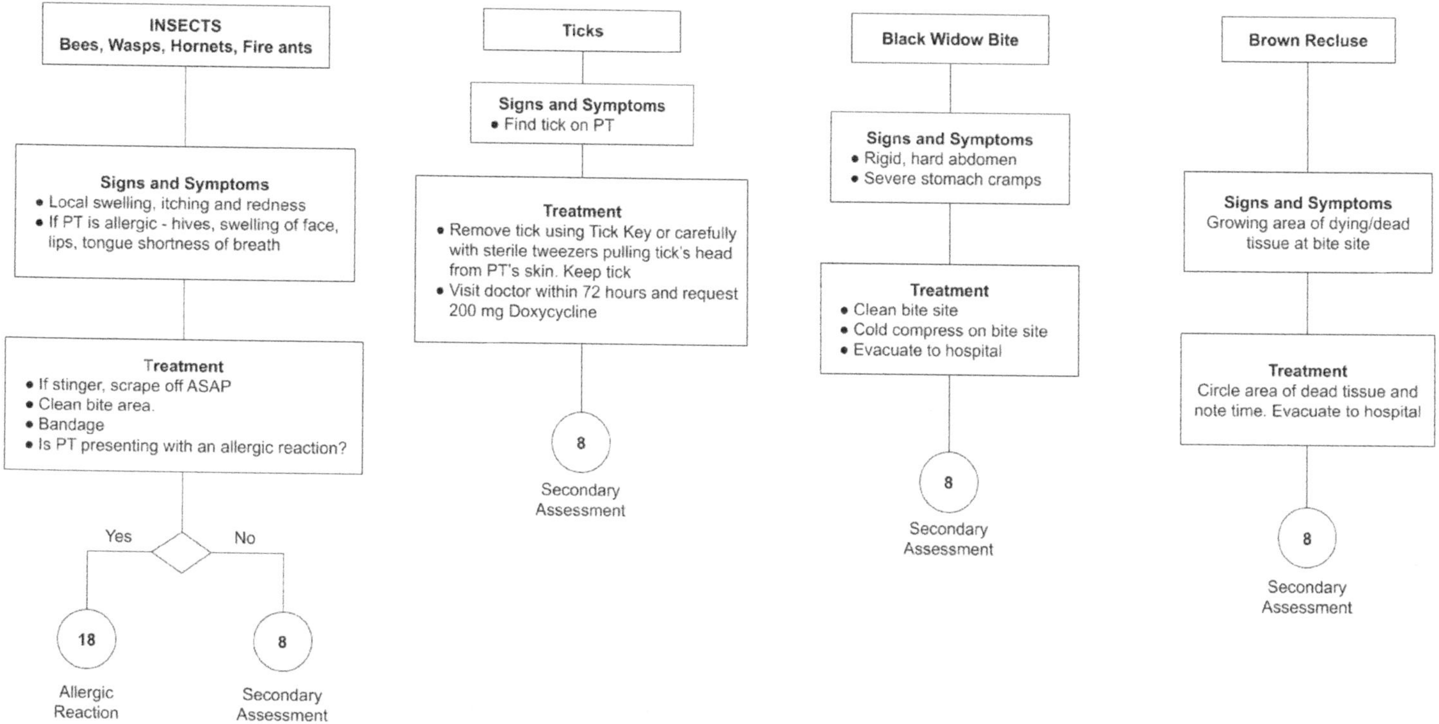

General Signs and Symptoms

- Two puncture wounds and possibly one of more of the following:
  - Swelling and redness around the wounds
  - Pain at the bite site
  - Difficulty breathing
  - Vomiting and nausea
  - Blurred vision
  - Sweating and salivating
  - Numbness in the face and limbs

Treatment

- Remove constricting items
- Clean and bandage
- If extremity, immobilize below heart
- Keep PT calm
- If are safely able, capture a photo of the snake
- Evacuate the PT to hospital immediately. The patient should not walk unless it is unavoidable for evacuation.

8 **Secondary Assessment**

BURNS

1st Degree Burn

Signs and Symptoms
- Red
- Hot
- Tender

Treatment
- Remove heat source.
- Remove area clothing
- Remove constricting items and jewelry
- Immediately cool - flowing water - for 15 minutes
- Clean
- 100% Aloe
- Moist sterile dressing

2nd Degree Burn

Signs and Symptoms
- 1st degree S/S plus:
- Swelling
- Blisters appear

Treatment
- 1st degree TX plus:
- Don't pop blister
- If the burn area is greater than the size of PT's palm - evacuate to hospital

3rd Degree Burn

Signs and Symptoms
- Charred - or -
- White like steamed chicken
- No pain at burn site

Treatment
LIFE THREAT
- 1st and 2nd degree TX plus:
- Remove heat source
- Dry sterile gauze
- Seal with plastic
- Hydrate and feed patient
- Watch for hypothermia
- Evacuate PT to hospital

8 Secondary Assessment

Chemical Burns
- Dry Chemicals - Brush away the chemical from the PT's skin. Flush the PT's skin with water for 15 minutes.
- Wet Chemicals - Flush the PT's skin with water for 15 minutes.

FROST BITE

1st Degree Frostbite

Signs and Symptoms
- Numb
- Cold
- White/Waxy
- Malleable

Treatment
- Remove jewelry
- Field re-warm: skin-to-skin
- Warm rest of PT's body
- Do not massage

2nd Degree Frostbite

Signs and Symptoms
- 1st degree S/S
- Bleb (Blister)
- Discoloration

Treatment
- 1st degree TX plus:
- Don't pop bleb
- Beware of refreezing
- Evacuate PT to hospital

3rd Degree Frostbite

Signs and Symptoms
- Numb
- Cold
- White
- Rock hard

Treatment
- Do not re-warm the affected body part in the field
- Protect body part
- Watch for hypothermia.
- Evacuate PT to hospital

8

Secondary Assessment

Acute Mountain Sickness (AMS)

Signs and Symptoms
- Headache plus any of following:
- Sleeping difficulty
- Fatigue
- Dizziness
- Loss of appetite
- Nausea
- Vomiting

Treatment
- Descend 2K - 3K Feet
- Rest and acclimatize
- Hydrate and feed
- Oxygen if available
- Descend further if no improvement in 12-24 hours and seek medical attention

High Altitude Pulmonary Edema (HAPE)

Signs and Symptoms
- AMS S/S plus any of the following
- Shortness of breath
- Coughing
- Chest pressure
- Breathing sounds - Crackles

Treatment
- Immediately descend 2k - 3k feet
- Oxygen or pressure chamber
- Hydrate
- Seek medication
- Evacuate to hospital

High Altitude Cerebral Edema (HACE)

Signs and Symptoms
- AMS S/S plus any of the following
- Confusion - inability to think or problem solve
- Hallucination

Treatment
- Immediately descend 2k - 3k feet
- Oxygen or pressure chamber
- Hydrate
- Seek medication
- Evacuate to hospital

8
Secondary Assessment

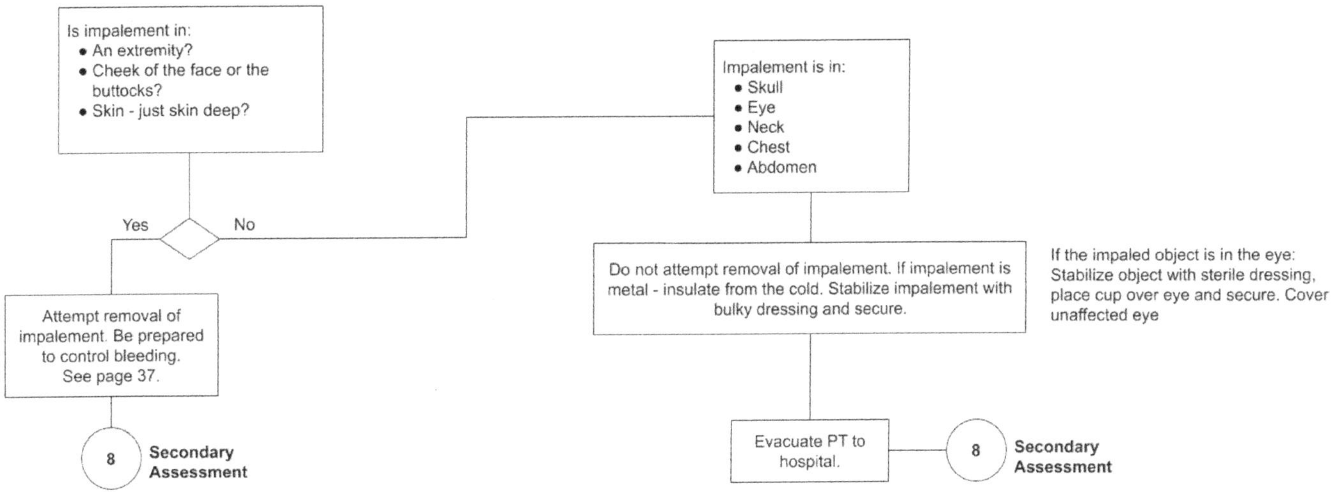
Is impalement in:
• An extremity?
• Cheek of the face or the buttocks?
• Skin - just skin deep?
Yes
No
Attempt removal of impalement. Be prepared to control bleeding. See page 37.
8
Secondary Assessment
Impalement is in:
• Skull
• Eye
• Neck
• Chest
• Abdomen
Do not attempt removal of impalement. If impalement is metal - insulate from the cold. Stabilize impalement with bulky dressing and secure.
If the impaled object is in the eye: Stabilize object with sterile dressing, place cup over eye and secure. Cover unaffected eye
Evacuate PT to hospital.
8
Secondary Assessment

LIGHTNING INJURIES

36

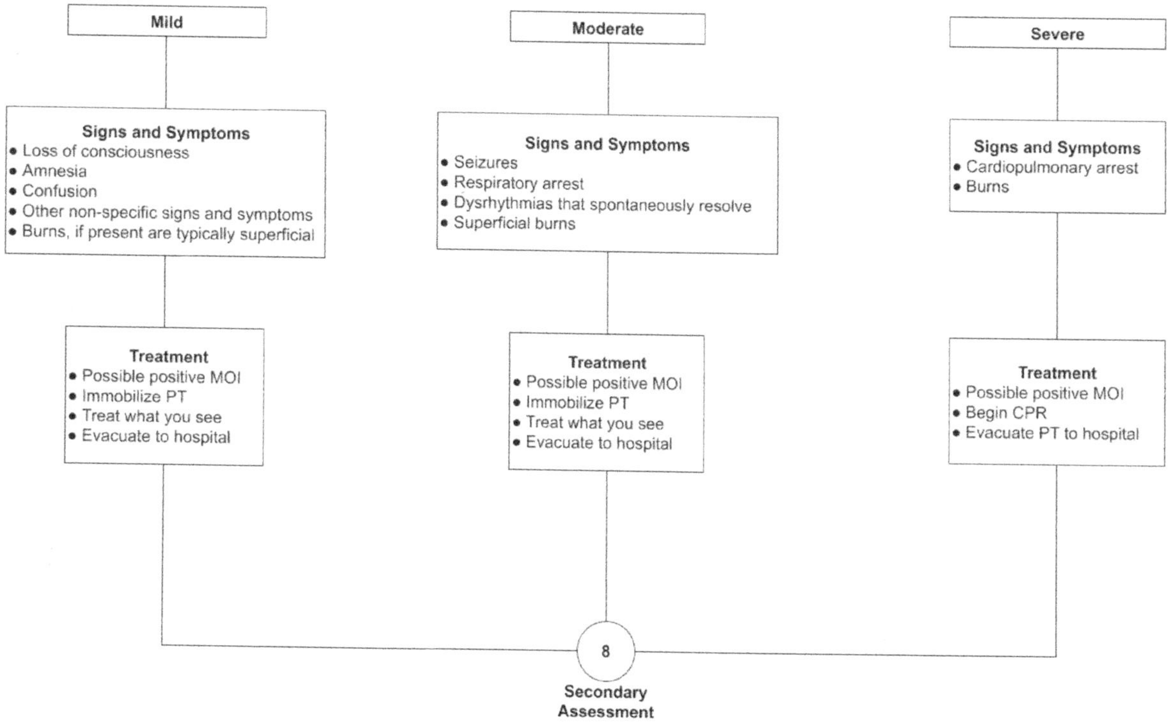

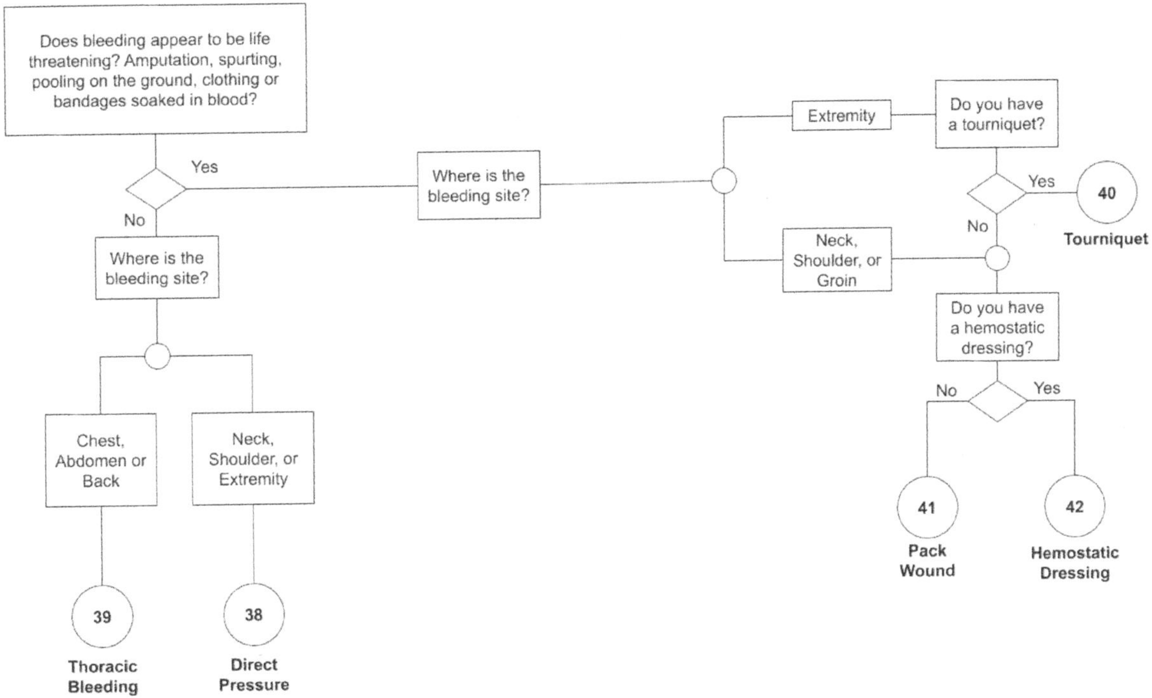
Does bleeding appear to be life threatening? Amputation, spurting, pooling on the ground, clothing or bandages soaked in blood?
Yes
No
Where is the bleeding site?
Where is the bleeding site?
Chest, Abdomen or Back
Neck, Shoulder, or Extremity
39
Thoracic Bleeding
38
Direct Pressure
Extremity
Do you have a tourniquet?
Yes
40
Tourniquet
No
Neck, Shoulder, or Groin
Do you have a hemostatic dressing?
No
Yes
41
Pack Wound
42
Hemostatic Dressing

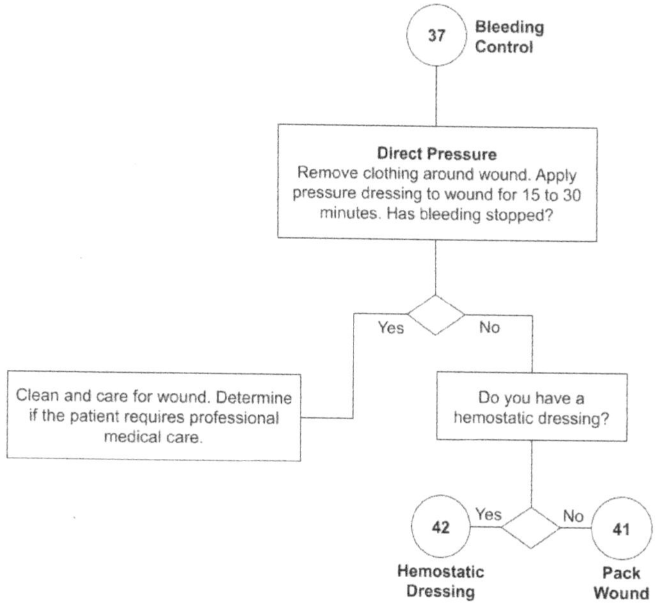
37
Bleeding Control
Direct Pressure
Remove clothing around wound. Apply pressure dressing to wound for 15 to 30 minutes. Has bleeding stopped?
Yes
No
Clean and care for wound. Determine if the patient requires professional medical care.
Do you have a hemostatic dressing?
Yes
No
42
Hemostatic Dressing
41
Pack Wound

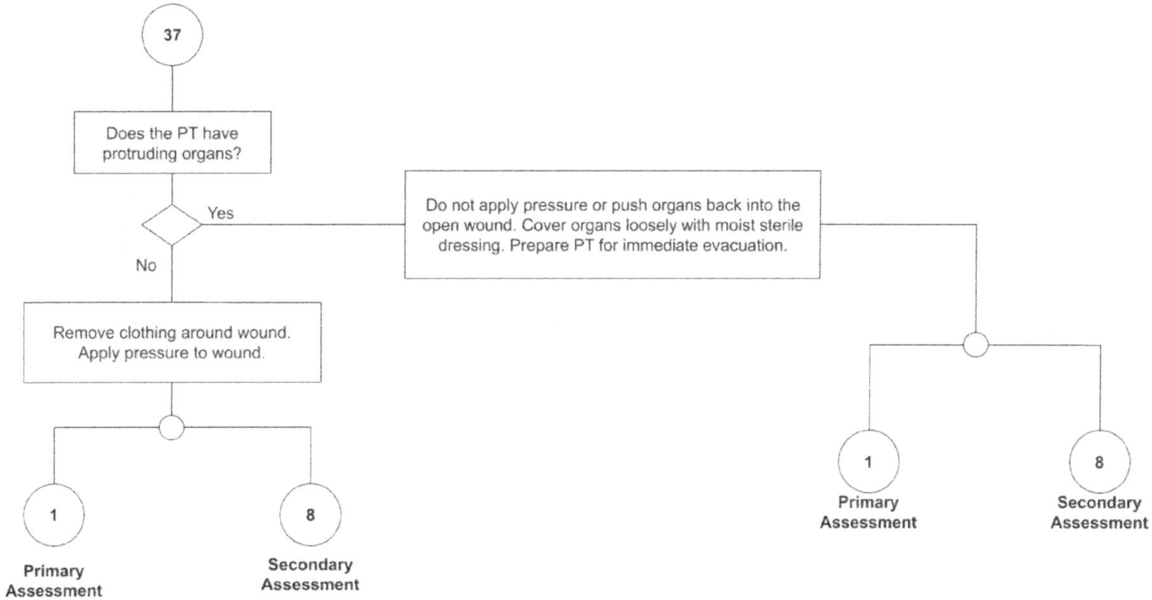
37
Does the PT have protruding organs?
Yes
Do not apply pressure or push organs back into the open wound. Cover organs loosely with moist sterile dressing. Prepare PT for immediate evacuation.
No
Remove clothing around wound. Apply pressure to wound.
1
Primary Assessment
8
Secondary Assessment
1
Primary Assessment
8
Secondary Assessment

BLEEDING CONTROL TOURNIQUET

LIFE THREAT

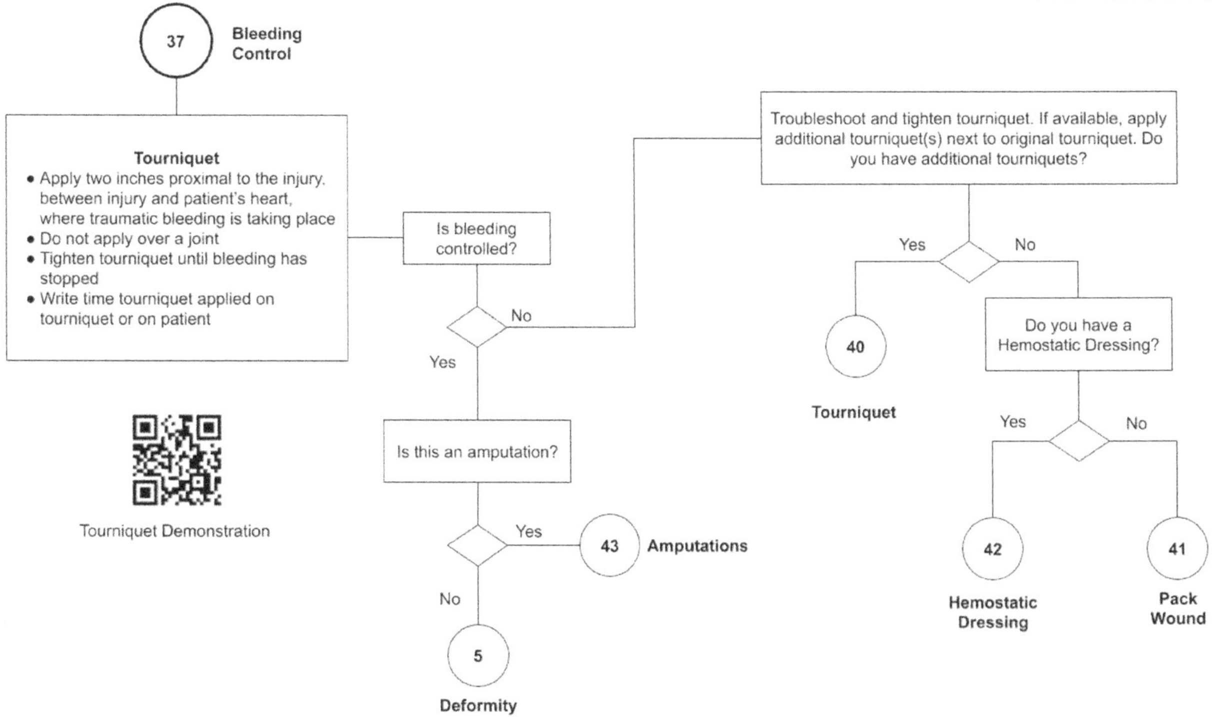

Bleeding Control
37

Tourniquet
40

Pack Wound
- Remove clothing from bleeding site.
- Wipe away any pooled blood
- Pack the wound with gauze.
- Apply steady pressure with both hands directly on top of the bleeding wound.
- Push down as hard as you are able.
- Hold pressure to stop bleeding.
- Continue pressure until bleeding has stopped or you are relieved by medical responders.

Wound Packing Demonstration

Is this an amputation?

Yes
43 Amputations

No
5 Deformity
1 Primary Assessment
8 Secondary Assessment

Alternative Bleeding Control Methods

- Digital Pressure - Push your gloved finger or thumb into wound, find the bleeding vessel and press it hard against bone.
- Find and and pinch close the bleeding vessel between your gloved forefinger and thumb.

Digital Pressure Demonstration

Digital Pinch Demonstration

BLEEDING CONTROL HEMOSTATIC DRESSING

LIFE THREAT

Bleeding Control (37) — Tourniquet (40)

Hemostatic Dressing

- Remove clothing from bleeding site.
- Wipe away any pooled blood
- Pack the wound with a hemostatic dressing.
- Apply steady pressure with both hands directly on top of the bleeding wound.
- Push down as hard as you are able for three minutes.
- Hold continuous pressure for 3 minutes.
- Reassess to ensure bleeding is controlled.
- Apply second gauze used if initial application fails to stop bleeding.
- Leave dressing in place and secure with bandage.
- Reassess frequently to monitor for recurrent bleeding.
- Evacuate PT to hospital immediately.

Hemostatic Dressing Demonstration

Is this an amputation?

- Yes → 43 Amputations
- No → 5 Deformity; 1 Primary Assessment; 8 Secondary Assessment

Alternative Bleeding Control Methods

- Digital Pressure - Push your gloved finger or thumb into wound, find the bleeding vessel and press it hard against bone.
- Find and and pinch close the bleeding vessel between your gloved forefinger and thumb.

Digital Pressure Demonstration

Digital Pinch Demonstration

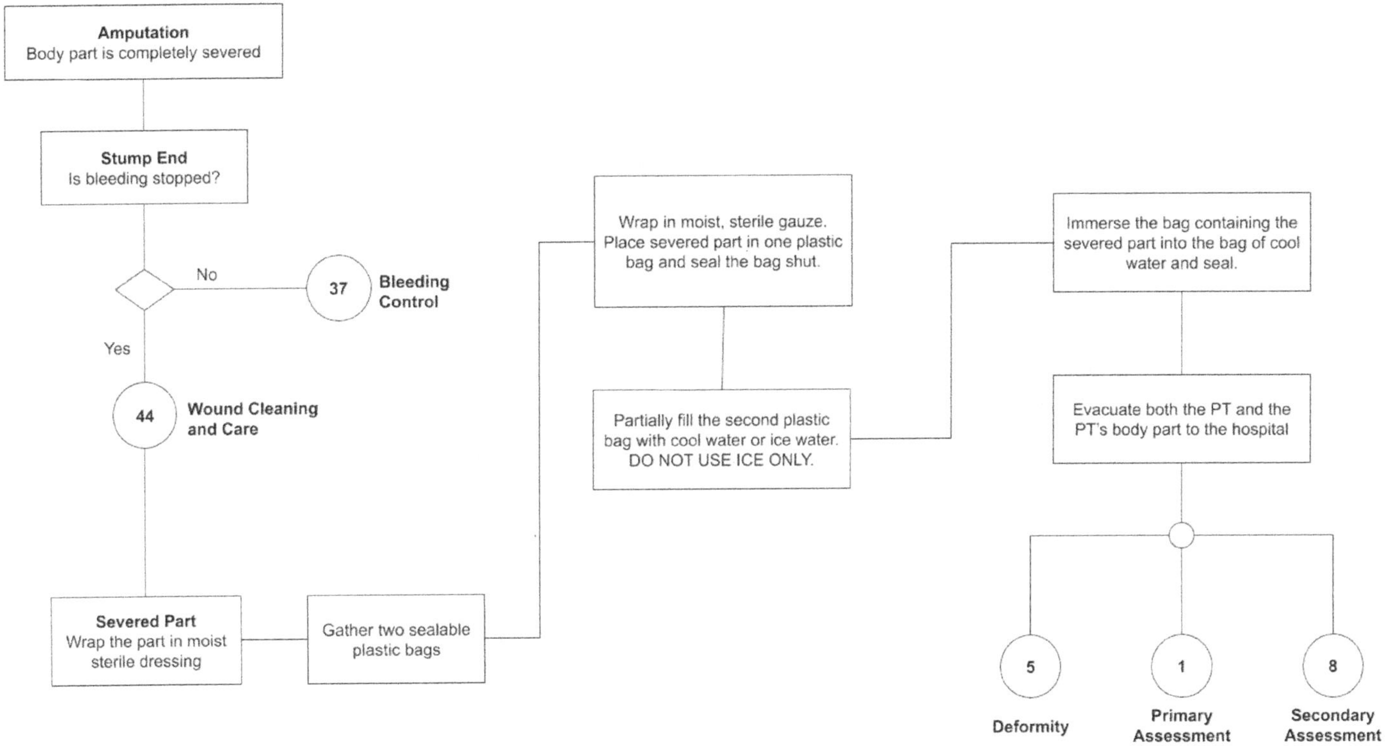
Amputation
Body part is completely severed
Stump End
Is bleeding stopped?
No
37
Bleeding Control
Yes
44
Wound Cleaning and Care
Severed Part
Wrap the part in moist sterile dressing
Gather two sealable plastic bags
Wrap in moist, sterile gauze. Place severed part in one plastic bag and seal the bag shut.
Partially fill the second plastic bag with cool water or ice water. DO NOT USE ICE ONLY.
Immerse the bag containing the severed part into the bag of cool water and seal.
Evacuate both the PT and the PT's body part to the hospital
5
Deformity
1
Primary Assessment
8
Secondary Assessment

WOUND CLEANING AND CARE

44

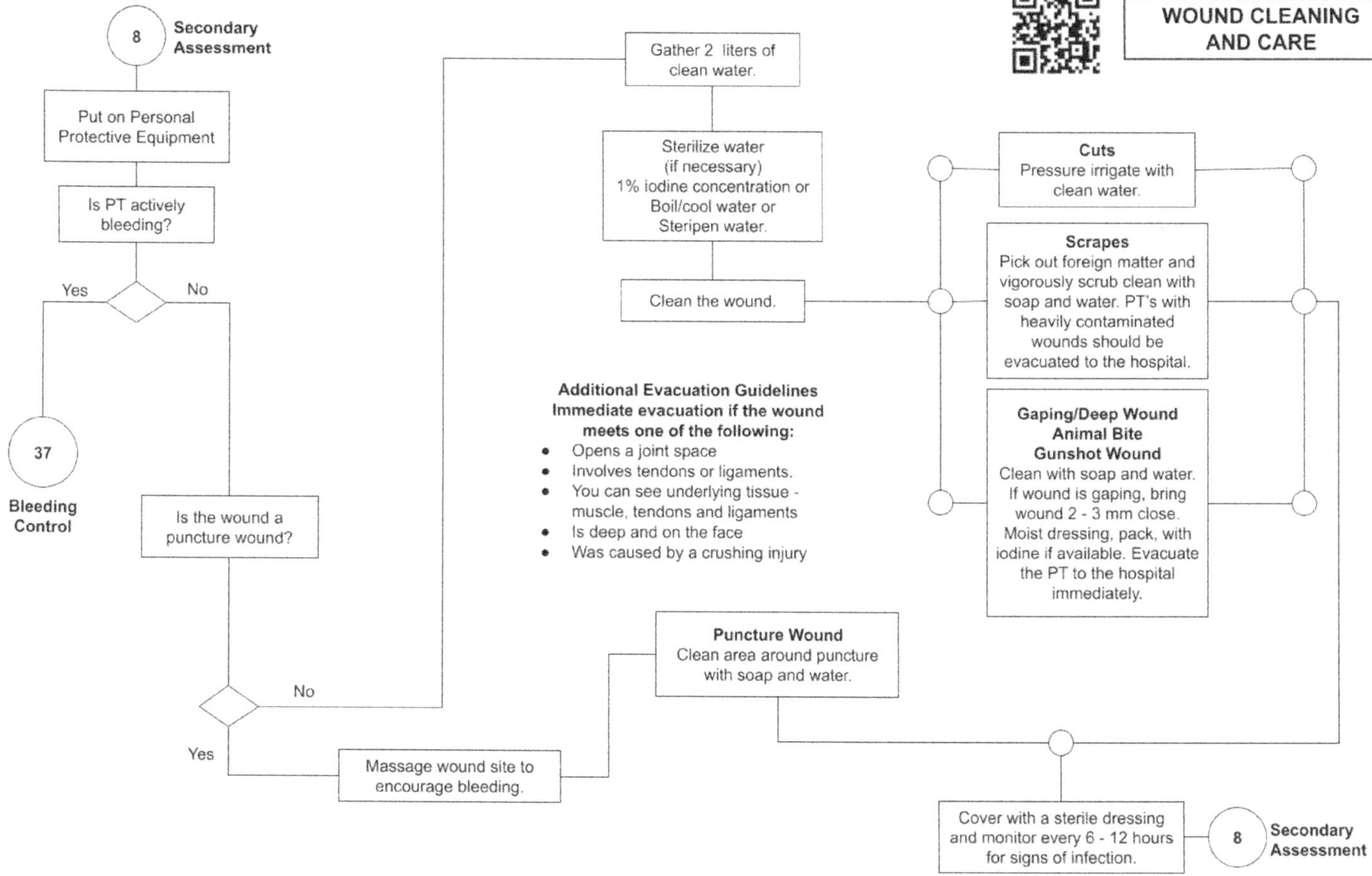

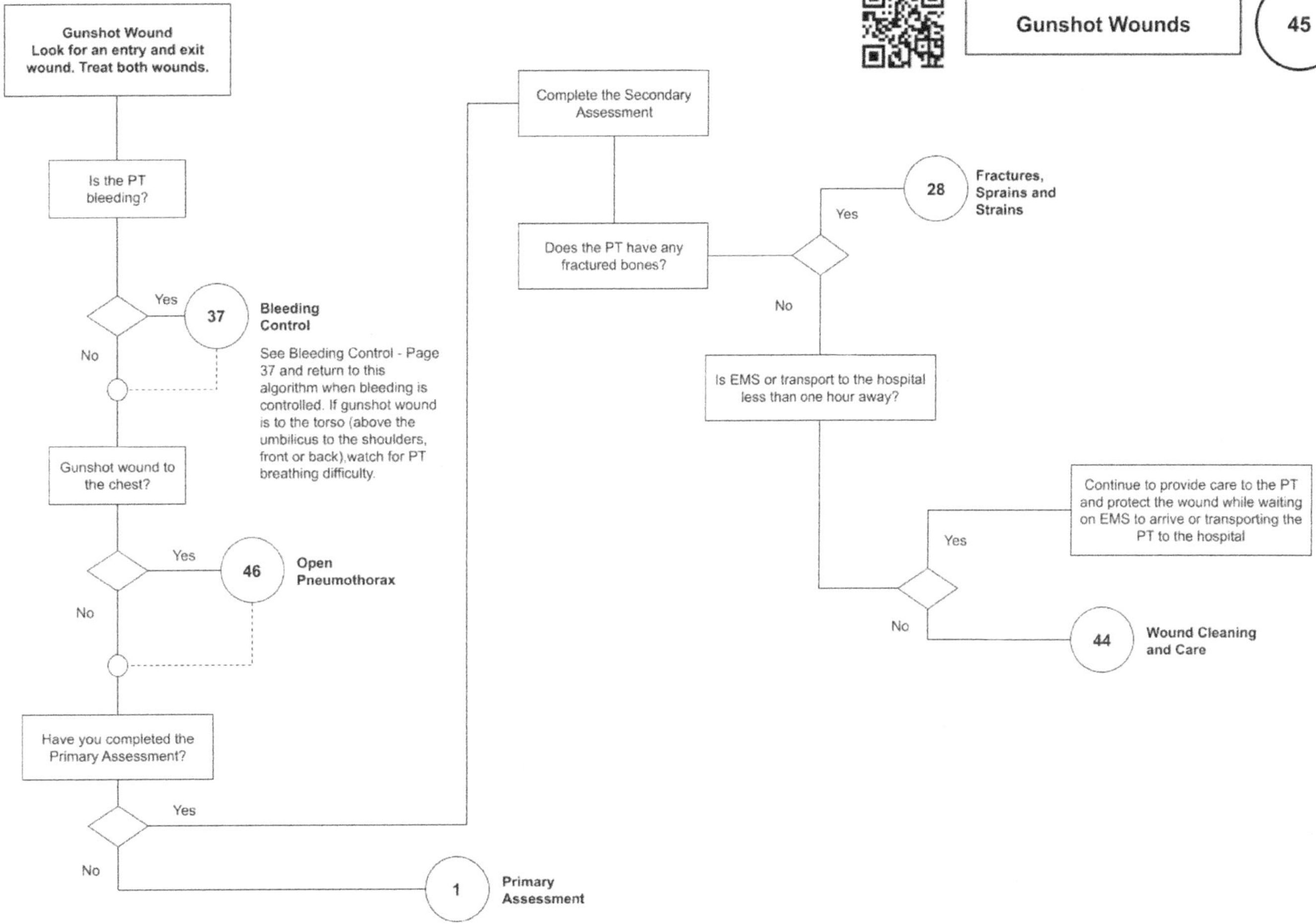
Gunshot Wound
Look for an entry and exit wound. Treat both wounds.
Is the PT bleeding?
Yes
37
Bleeding Control
See Bleeding Control - Page 37 and return to this algorithm when bleeding is controlled. If gunshot wound is to the torso (above the umbilicus to the shoulders, front or back),watch for PT breathing difficulty.
No
Gunshot wound to the chest?
Yes
46
Open Pneumothorax
No
Have you completed the Primary Assessment?
Yes
No
1
Primary Assessment
Complete the Secondary Assessment
Does the PT have any fractured bones?
Yes
28
Fractures, Sprains and Strains
No
Is EMS or transport to the hospital less than one hour away?
Yes
Continue to provide care to the PT and protect the wound while waiting on EMS to arrive or transporting the PT to the hospital
No
44
Wound Cleaning and Care

Open Pneumothorax

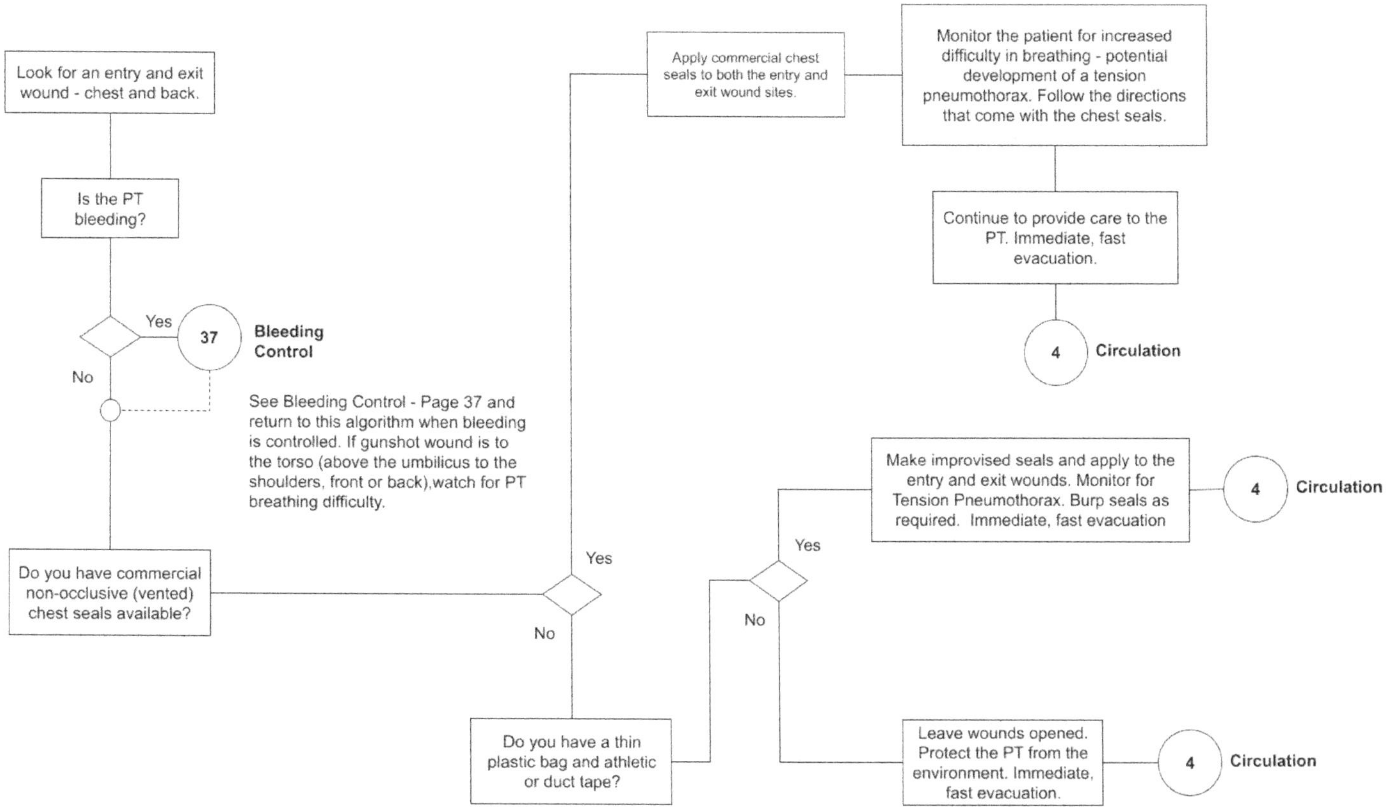

Meningitis Signs and Symptoms

- Fever (~100% cases)
- Headache (>90% cases)
- Stiff Neck (Most all cases)
- Petechial Rash (>50% cases)
- Mental Confusion (if Bacterial Meningitis)

Other Signs to Look For:

- Kernig's Sign
- Brudzinski's Sign
- Seizures
- See Page 11B - Viral and Bacterial Illnesses

Do you suspect meningitis?

Yes: PT requires immediate evacuation to the hospital

No: 8 **Secondary Assessment**

LIFE THREAT

Meningitis Facts

- Incubation Period
  - 3 to 4 days
- Common in young adults living in close quarters
- Abrupt Onset
  - A few hours
- Fatality Rate
  - 9% - 12%

Stroke Signs and Symptoms

- Sudden numbness or weakness of face, arm, or leg, especially on one side of the body
- Sudden confusion, trouble speaking or understanding speech
- Sudden trouble seeing in one or both eyes
- Sudden trouble walking, dizziness, loss of balance or coordination
- Sudden sever headache with no known cause

Stroke FAST Acronym

Face Drooping - Look for drooping or numbness on one side of he face. Ask the PT to smile to make the droop more apparent.

Arm Weekness - Look for muscle weakness on one side of he body. Ask the person to raise both arms up and hold them for a count of ten. If one arm falls or begins to drop, then this could be a sign of a stroke.

Speech Difficulty - Is speech slurred? Is the person unable to speak or hard to understand? Ask the person to repeat a simple sentence.

Time - If the PT presents with any of these signs and symptoms, even if the signs ans symptoms go away, they require immediate transport to the hsopital.

PT requires immediate evacuation to the hospital

- AVPU - Alert, Verbal, Pain, Unresponsive
- BP = Blood Pressure
- C/C - Chief Complaint
- CSF - Cerebrospinal Fluid
- CSM - Circulation, Sensation, Motion
- HR = Heart Rate
- HX = History
- LOC = Level of Consciousness
- LLQ = Left Lower Quadrant - Abdomen
- LUQ = Left Upper Quadrant - Abdomen
- MOI = Mechanism of Injury
- PCC = Pale, Cool, Clammy
- PWD = Pink, Warm, Dry
- PAS = Patient Assessment System
- PPE - Personal Protective Equipment (See BSI)
- PT - Patient
- RICE = Rest, Ice, Compression, Elevation
- RLQ = Right Lower Quadrant - Abdomen
- RUQ = Right Upper Quadrant - Abdomen
- RR = Respiratory Rate
- S/S = Signs and Symptoms
- SAMPLE - Signs/Symptoms, Allergies, Medications, Past Medical History, Last oral intake, last urinary and rectal output, Events leading up to crisis
- SOAP = Subjective, Objective, Assessment, Plan
- TX = Treatment
- WFA = Wilderness First Aid

SOAP NOTE

50

Subjective: (Age, Sex, MOI, NOI, Chief Complaint)

Objective: Vital signs, patient exam, SAMPLE history

Signs and Symptoms:

Allergies:

Medications:

Past pertinent medical history:

Last in and out:

Events leading up to accident:

Patient Exam: Describe the location of pain, tenderness and injuries:

VITAL SIGNS				
Time				
RR & Effort				
HR and Effort				
LOC - A&O x ?				
Skin - C, T, M				

Assessment: (Problem List)

Plan: (Plan for each problem on the problem list)

Monitor - How often do you plan to monitor the patient?

Rescue Plan:

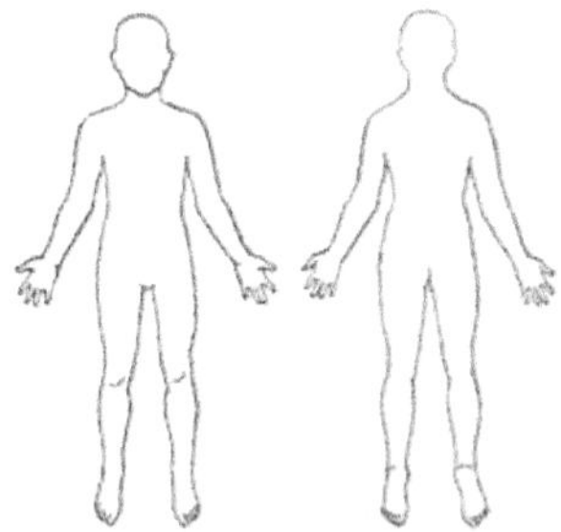

Sources – 51

AN EVIDENCE-BASED PREHOSPITAL GUIDELINE FOR EXTERNAL HEMORRHAGE CONTROL: AMERICAN COLLEGE OF SURGEONS COMMITTEE ON TRAUMA. (2014, May 18). Retrieved from https://www.facs.org/~/media/files/quality programs/trauma/education/acscot evidencebased prehospital guidelines for external hemmorrhage control.ashx

Auerbach, Paul S. Medicine for the Outdoors: The Essential Guide to Emergency Medical Procedures and First Aid. London: Elsevier Health Sciences, 2009.

Austere emergency medical support (AEMS) field guide. (n.d.). Retrieved October 4, 2021, from https://www.amr.net/solutions/federal-disaster-response-team/references-and-resources/dhs-austere-ems-field-guide.pdf.

Davis, Chris, Anna Engeln, Eric L. Johnson, Scott E. Mcintosh, Ken Zafren, Arthur A. Islas, Christopher Mcstay, William R. Smith, and Tracy Cushing. "Wilderness Medical Society Practice Guidelines for the Prevention and Treatment of Lightning Injuries: 2014 Update." Wilderness & Environmental Medicine 25, no. 4 (2014). https://doi.org/10.1016/j.wem.2014.08.011.

Dow, Jennifer, Gordon G. Giesbrecht, Daniel F. Danzl, Hermann Brugger, Emily B. Sagalyn, Beat Walpoth, Paul S. Auerbach, et al. "Wilderness Medical Society Clinical Practice Guidelines for the Out-of-Hospital Evaluation and Treatment of Accidental Hypothermia: 2019 Update." Wilderness & Environmental Medicine 30, no. 4 (2019). https://doi.org/10.1016/j.wem.2019.10.002.

Hawkins, Seth C., Jason Williams, Brad L. Bennett, Arthur Islas, Dietrich Whitfield Kayser, and Robert Quinn. "Wilderness Medical Society Clinical Practice Guidelines for Spinal Cord Protection." Wilderness & Environmental Medicine 30, no. 4 (2019). https://doi.org/10.1016/j.wem.2019.08.001.

Hubbell, F. (2014). Wildcare: Working in less than desirable conditions and remote environments. Conway, NH: TMC Books/Stonehearth Open Learning Opportunities.

Isaac, J. (2013). Outward Bound wilderness first-aid handbook. Guilford, CT: Globe Pequot Press.

Lipman, Grant S., Kurt P. Eifling, Mark A. Ellis, Flavio G. Gaudio, Edward M. Otten, and Colin K. Grissom. "Wilderness Medical Society Practice Guidelines for the Prevention and Treatment of Heat-Related Illness: 2014 Update." Wilderness & Environmental Medicine 25, no. 4 (2014). https://doi.org/10.1016/j.wem.2014.07.017.

Luks, Andrew M., Paul S. Auerbach, Luanne Freer, Colin K. Grissom, Linda E. Keyes, Scott E. Mcintosh, George W. Rodway, Robert B. Schoene, Ken Zafren, and Peter H. Hackett. "Wilderness Medical Society Clinical Practice Guidelines for the Prevention and Treatment of Acute Altitude Illness: 2019 Update." Wilderness & Environmental Medicine 30, no. 4 (2019). https://doi.org/10.1016/j.wem.2019.04.006.

Mcintosh, Scott E., Matthew Opacic, Luanne Freer, Colin K. Grissom, Paul S. Auerbach, George W. Rodway, Amalia Cochran, et al. "Wilderness Medical Society Practice Guidelines for the Prevention and Treatment of Frostbite: 2014 Update." Wilderness & Environmental Medicine 25, no. 4 (2014). https://doi.org/10.1016/j.wem.2014.09.001.

NAEMT. (2016). PHTLS: Prehospital trauma life support (8th ed.). S.l.: JONES & BARTLETT LEARNING.

Pollak, A. N., Edgerly, D., McKenna, K., & Vitberg, D. A. (2017). Emergency care and transportation of the sick and injured (11th ed.). Burlington, MA: Jones & Bartlett Learning.

Quinn, Robert H., Ian Wedmore, Eric L. Johnson, Arthur A. Islas, Anne Anglim, Ken Zafren, Cindy Bitter, and Vicki Mazzorana. "Wilderness Medical Society Practice Guidelines for Basic Wound Management in the Austere Environment: 2014 Update." Wilderness & Environmental Medicine 25, no. 4 (2014). https://doi.org/10.1016/j.wem.2014.08.015.

Riot medicine. Riot Medicine. (n.d.). Retrieved October 4, 2020, from https://riotmedicine.net/.

Schimelpfenig, T., & Safford, J. M. (2016). NOLS wilderness medicine. Lanham, MD: Stackpole Books.

Scope and Guidelines 2019. Wilderness Medicine Education Cooperative - WFA. (n.d.). Retrieved October 4, 2021, from https://www.wildmededucationcollaborative.org/scope-of-practice-documents.html and https://wildsafety.com/WMS/WFA-SOP.pdf

Thygerson, A. L., Thygerson, S. M., Thygerson, J. S., Backer, H. D., Bowman, W. D., Paton, B. C., . . . Backer, H. D. (2019). Wilderness first aid: Emergency care in remote locations. Burlington, MA: Jones & Bartlett Learning.

Wilderness First Aid Curriculum ... - Boy Scouts of America. (n.d.). Retrieved October 4, 2021, from https://filestore.scouting.org/filestore/pdf/680-008.pdf.